Beyond the Treadmill

A Christian perspective
on pressure and stress

Rowland Moss

Scripture Union
130 City Road, London EC1V 2NJ

ISBN 0 86201 381 X

Phototypeset by Input Typesetting Ltd, London.
Printed and bound in Great Britain
by Cox and Wyman Ltd, Reading.

Contents

	page
Preface	5
Foreword	7
A personal experience	9

PART ONE
Rat race in a cage

The contemporary scene	19
1 Pressures at work	21
2 Pressures in society	30
3 Pressures in the church	41
4 Stop the mill; I want to get off!	54

PART TWO
The view from outside the cage

5 Blindness in the cage	63
6 The results of worldly blindness	68
7 The symptoms of worldly blindness	73

PART THREE
In the race but not the cage

| 8 Sharing God's view | 81 |
| 9 Sharing with the people of God | 92 |

PART FOUR
Turning the treadmill into a ladder

10	Under pressure in the Old Testament	105
11	Under pressure in the New Testament	119
12	Practical actions	129

PART FIVE
Broken by the mill

13	Self-help for the broken	149
14	Helping the broken	161
15	Helping non-Christians and lapsed Christians	169

Epilogue	173
Further reading	180
Appendix A: Sunday worship	185
Appendix B: Towards a personal check-up	187

Preface

This book is not a dispassionate analysis of the problems of pressure and stress in the society in which we live. Nor could it be. Coming to breaking-point when pressure and stress become intolerable is an experience of such trauma that objective consideration is no longer possible. I doubt that anyone who can write with clinical precision on these matters has really been to the depths which complete breakdown involves. Nor is this a book which sets out a series of steps by which depression and breakdown can be conquered or avoided altogether. I merely offer these reflections ten years after the event, when perhaps a wider and deeper view is possible, in order to help both those who suffer now and those who are perhaps, all unknown to themselves, heading towards breaking-point.

Depression and breakdown are intensely personal and isolating experiences. Each one who comes to that point needs equally personal and individual attention in order to come through. Renewal and refreshment can always be the outcome if we suffer patiently, persevere and seek to learn from the experience by the guidance of God by his Spirit through the scriptures. Its bitterness can then be transformed into unspeakable joy in more fruitful service.

I am grateful to my bishop, the Right Reverend Michael Baughen, for writing the foreword; to Becky Totterdell, a patient and perceptive editor, for working so hard on the first draft, and posing so many perceptive questions; to my wife, Sheena, my family and friends who stood by me in the darkness; and above all to my Lord for leading me into and bringing me through the valley of the dark shadow that can be touched. My thanks are beyond words. There is therefore no more to say!

Rowland Moss
Cheadle Hulme, Cheshire

Foreword

If we are about to enter hospital for an operation, it is not the assuring words of the surgeon or medical staff that help us most, but the words of those who have already had the operation – they know what it is *really* like.

Rowland Moss knows what it is *really* like to have a complete breakdown, with all the darkness of depression overwhelming him; he also has come out of it to a leading position in the academic world and to ordained ministry. We know he knows as we begin the book and find ourselves gripped by the vivid account of his own breakdown. This is followed by the highly effective parable of the cage, the treadmill and the ladder.

Yet our reading of the book cannot be just out of interest. Here is straight talking, warning and advice which needs to be taken on board by every church member – and particularly by evangelical Christians because of the very high level of activity in evangelical churches. The taking on of more and more activities can so frequently result in an inability to take on *any* activity. Professor Moss shows us that stress and strain can actually be compounded by Christian activity.

I most warmly commend this book to every Christian worker. It is written by a talented, senior Christian, who is also ordained and serves in my Diocese of Chester with expertise and love. Prevention is far, far better than cure. This book is preventive medicine. How strongly I agree with Rowland Moss that worship and prayer, spiritual reality and the maturing of our love-union with Christ is the vital centre for churches and Christians. All activity is secondary to this. Christ says to each of us what he said to Peter: 'Do you love me?'

This book may make you put on some brakes but avoid your breaking. God help you to read and respond – for his glory.

Michael Baughen
Bishop of Chester

7

A personal experience

Suddenly the tropical sun became an agony. I broke out in a cold sweat. I turned to make my way back along the beach to my room in the hotel. As I climbed the dunes I became unbearably dizzy and light-headed. I scarcely made it back to my room before I passed out on the bed in a peculiar semi-faint. In painful half-consciousness I became aware of my heart doing strange things – palpitations getting stronger, then passing into a rapidly accelerating beat, then stopping, followed by a complete loss of consciousness as the whole room spun. Then, semi-conscious again, the cycle was repeated, with developing nausea; then again; and again; and again; and again; I do not know how many times. And each time the contrast between the vibrating and accelerating spasms of my heart, and the subsequent silence and unconsciousness, became more striking. As the room rotated, I seemed to float above the bed. I was aware that what I had thought were palpitations were not; they were quite different and much more violent and deep. Subsequently they were diagnosed as very severe fibrillation.

I was alone. There was no real prospect of my moving, still less of anyone coming to my room; no possibility of ringing for help; no contact with anyone. As the symptoms worsened with each cycle, I became more and more convinced that death was near and inevitable, for I could not believe that my heart could continue to sustain such violent spasms for long without collapse. I committed myself to the Lord, and I seemed to hover continually at the brink of time, with part of me at the entrance to eternity, and the rest still anchored to the earth, to place and time. I knew no fear. I was glad to accept the call of the Lord to himself in that hotel room in Tanzania, 5,000 miles from home, my family, my dearest friends.

Then, miraculously as I now believe, the cycles ceased. I do not know how long they continued. I lay on the bed pouring perspiration, conscious only of the chill of a high temperature and the now steady beat of my heart. I lay motionless for hours, until there was a knock on the door. Two other long-term visitors to the university had missed me at dinner, and had come to find out why I was not present in our usual group.

It was 10 pm. I had felt unwell while walking along the shore at about 1.30 pm – adequately protected from the sun!

The medical officer from Dar es Salaam was summoned, and, after examining me, diagnosed malaria and pumped me full of chloroquine. I was too ill, and insufficiently conscious, to describe adequately the symptoms surrounding the cycles of the afternoon, even though he was puzzled by my high blood pressure. One of the other visitors moved into the spare bed in the room overnight, to keep an eye on me.

The next morning I was completely washed out, but

lucid – and a different person. I was continually conscious of the beat of my heart, now back to normal; I was unable to eat, for my stomach was too tense and knotted; I was prone to abject panic at the least problem.

During the next few days, though I managed to get back to the university to complete my teaching commitment, I developed a physical horror of the room in which I was staying, and, to a lesser degree, of the whole hotel.

Worst of all, I could not sleep, even with aid of substantial doses of phenobarbitone. More chloroquine was administered, and my blood pressure stayed high despite the administration of a strong drug to reduce it.

After ten days it was decided that I should return to Britain as soon as possible. Since I had completed my teaching commitment, all I would miss would be the three weeks of up-country visits which had been planned as a climax to my visit.

So the two kind Christian friends – one British, the other Tanzanian – who had so graciously taken me in to their small flat on the university campus to relieve me of the pressure of living in the hotel, put me on the plane to London, after twelve hours' delay and two visits to the airport.

As soon as the plane took off after its brief stop at Nairobi, on its non-stop flight to London, my whole mind and body relaxed and I slept peacefully for the first time in a fortnight. After waking up, I ate my first substantial meal in the same period – and developed severe indigestion as a result!

At Heathrow I was too weak to walk through Immigration and Customs, and I was wheeled through the usual formalities in a wheelchair, which had been radioed for by the sympathetic British Airways captain. I was met by a family whose faces could not hide their deep shock at my appearance, so great was the transformation from seven weeks before. I had lost two stone in weight – in other circumstances no bad thing! And my hair had turned grey in the short space of two weeks.

These events were a watershed in my experience. They were the beginning of three years of chronic stress and depression; and, as I now realize, the culmination of several years of growing pressure and strain in every area of my life. They were possibly triggered by some mysterious tropical virus, though none was detected on my return home; exhaustive cardiac examinations revealed no heart disease or damage.

After my return home I began gradually to improve in health, though with the persistent recurrence of stress symptoms at the slightest extra pressure. I resumed my responsibilities at Birmingham University after several weeks' rest, but as the summer of 1975 passed into autumn, and on into winter, the stress symptoms continued, and I became more and more depressed. I continued my work at the university and in church only with the aid of drugs.

In 1976 the symptoms continued and I was sinking deeper into depression. A great permanent cloud descended. Extra commitments in the middle of 1976 brought me once again close to breaking-point, and I was saved only by stronger drugs and sedatives. In the end I had to cut all my commitments and take three months off work – though my head of department insisted that I mark my examination scripts!

By the end of that year the stress symptoms had diminished, but the depression was much worse. I still panicked at the slightest crisis, and any stress produced clear symptoms – after the pressure had passed. Even the commitment to complete a scientific paper to a deadline could have an effect. I gave up playing the organ at church, which had always been a relaxing pleasure. Soon I was only managing to suffer one service of worship on a Sunday, when to go as often as possible had once been a chief delight.

In late 1976 and throughout 1977 I lived in a perpetual dark, clinging cloud. Life was an aimless walk in a dark and enervating, almost tangible, suffocating fog. I was oppressed and depressed by forces I could neither confront nor identify. The causes were always lurking around the next corner, but never there when I turned it.

Prayer was an empty discipline maintained by habit; worship a hollow act undertaken as an unpleasant duty. At the university my teaching became a taxing chore, research and writing an evil necessity, departmental and university committees (never a pleasure!) an implacable horror to be faced out with a stoical indifference. My memory began to deteriorate and, from a reasonably fluent argument delivered from outline notes with real interest and enthusiasm, my lectures became dull, monotonous readings from almost fully written-out scripts – a fact my students were not slow to comment on, somewhat forcefully!

I had no will to rise in the morning, and no motivation to engage in any activity, no enjoyment in any task, and no satisfaction in any project successfully completed. I wallowed in deepening despair. There was no real interaction with the present, still less any joy in the mercies of the past or any hope or promise for the future – only a dark shadow that could be felt.

At that point the word of the Lord met me. I had engaged in desultory Bible study, and I had turned some of my experience into poetry, the only catharsis which seemed to have any therapeutic influence. I became fascinated with the use in the Old Testament of the Hebrew word *tsalmaveth* – thick darkness, the darkness that can be touched, the valley of the shadow of death! Yes! the valley of the dark clinging shadow that can be touched! Yes! *my* shadow! It was a direct word of the Lord to me. Not that the depression lifted; the shadow was still there; but now I had a word of the Lord to hang on to. And I did, like grim death.

'Yea though I walk through the valley of the shadow that can be felt, I will fear no evil, *for Thou art with me*.' Words which I had known since childhood, which I had read dozens of times, which I knew by heart, now had meaning *for me personally*. God the Lord was *with me* – whether I felt it or not, whether conscious of his presence or not, whether I believed it or not; there were no conditions, just a straight statement of fact. I realized that all valleys, all dark defiles, have an end sooner or later; that eventually the path opens out into the light. Then the panorama of God's purpose spreads out before our eyes, and into the distance beyond the farthest reaches of our imagination. I had a hope to grasp at last.

The tormented psalmist knew this experience:

'Why are you cast down, O my soul,
  and why are you disquieted within me?
Hope in God; for I *shall* again praise him,
  my help and my God.'

(Ps 42:5,11; 43:5 RSV.)

And so did I – in my reason, in my acceptance of God's bare word.

The depression did not lift; it became worse, compounded by the death of my father, a saint of God to whom I had grown more and more close as he and I both became older. The dark shadow clung more closely, and still more closely, like a soaked, musty sack, until I felt enmeshed in it, unable to escape; I was stifled, suffocating in a sodden shroud.

In February 1978 I was at the complete end of myself; I could no longer continue the dishonest charade called my life – my career, my Christian work and commitment, my family responsibilities. In anger – yes, *anger*, born of desperation – I cried to the Lord, 'I can't go on! You have broken me! Finish the job and take away my life! I am no longer any use to you or to anyone!'

More composedly and rationally, I prayed, 'Lord, if you do not do something then I shall have to resign my chair at the university, and give up all my activities in the church of Christ. I cannot go on! I cannot stand it any longer!'

I was finished and completely broken. The Lord heard, and answered. The cloud lifted; within three days it had gone completely. Like the sun with morning mist, the light of the face of the Lord dissipated the dark shadow, at first slowly, them more rapidly, and then completely. The demons of the valley fled at his word, and their nauseating vapours went with them. The sunlight of the Lord's presence gradually revealed undreamt-of vistas of service, for deep spiritual renewal followed, and continued to grow as he led me into paths I could not have imagined, surrounded by lush green pastures.

The stress symptoms, which had been present throughout the depression, became less frequent and less severe and distressing, and eventually disappeared.

My deliverance from the depression, which occurred in late February, was the beginning of a process of physical, mental and spiritual rebuilding. The drugs were dispensed with completely by September, and in the early months of 1979 I was invited to the University of Salford, an invitation which, even three months earlier, I could not have considered. The move to the north-west of England led me into the Anglican Communion, and then into its ordained ministry, while still retaining full and increasing responsibilities in the university.

These experiences raise many questions. Do I regret them? No, for I learnt so much through them about myself, and about the Lord; maybe they were things I could not have learnt any other way.

Would my loving Lord have led me by such a hard path if I had been able to learn those lessons by any easier way? He knew what he wanted to make of me – and still does; and I can now share and sympathize with those who suffer the agonies of the valley now, in a way someone who has never experienced the dark, clinging, tangible cloud can never do. My valley of terror led out into the light. So did the psalmist's, and like him I have found at the outfall of the valley a rich banquet spread out to be enjoyed in the presence of those very enemies who harassed and numbed me with fear in the valley. Can that not be some small encouragement to the saints who are passing through the valley today?

Could the whole sequence of events have been avoided? Perhaps, had I been wiser – but I wasn't. Others might benefit from my foolishness.

Should Christians suffer from depression and stress? Is it sinful to be depressed? Whatever the answers to those two questions are, the fact remains that many Christians *do* suffer from depression, as the response I have had to the article from which this prologue is drawn so clearly indicates.

There are other questions too: Should Christians who suffer depression and stress expect and claim instant healing? Is it a lack of faith not to? After all, depression is a mental illness, not something physical, so isn't it different, and somehow more curable by spiritual therapy?

So now, ten years after the onset of my depression, the time has perhaps come to reflect biblically, and at some length, on some of these questions.

I cannot claim psychiatric expertise, but I now have a training in theology accepted by the Church of England! I write merely as a victim reflecting on an experience which comes to many Christians in this pressured society of ours; I can no longer speak with detached objectivity. I am one of the rats who fell exhausted off the treadmill – and thus learnt how to turn the treadmill into a ladder.

PART ONE

Rat race in a cage:

the contemporary scene

The contemporary scene

Have you ever watched a hamster on a treadmill? It spends a great deal of time and energy getting nowhere. It is supposed to enjoy it, though I have never had a close enough relationship with a hamster to find out. But the exercise is the substitute for the real thing, for in its life in the wild it would spend the energy in foraging for food and other activities. Because it is in a cage, the exercise is pointless.

We speak of 'the rat race', and accept it as a necessary part of life. For many of us, other human beings are rivals, even enemies, in the race to get to the top. We spend a great deal of energy in trying to put ourselves a step ahead. We are like rats on a treadmill striving for the elusive prize at the top, which we never reach. The only way of escape seems to be either to opt out or to fall off completely exhausted. Even if we reach the top, staying there takes even more effort and requires a delicate balancing act. The bitter irony is that eventually we all end up dead on the floor of the cage, however near the top of the mill we manage to get.

The treadmill is futile because it doesn't lead anywhere and *cannot* lead anywhere because it is set in a cage. If it were a ladder, and long enough, it would lead out of the cage. And yet a treadmill is simply a ladder bent into a circle so that its two ends meet and are joined. It is possible to turn a treadmill back into a ladder, but only if we are prepared to break out of the cage.

The cage of rats, fully equipped with numerous inviting treadmills, is a picture of the society in which we live. God intended the ladder to lead us to glory, but we have turned it into a treadmill which leads nowhere, because we have set our sights only on the goals we can see within the cage. Until we begin to see beyond the cage we shall never be able to turn our treadmill into a ladder. So, caught in the cage, we are stuck on the treadmill. Many non-Christians realize it, like the very successful academic who wrote:

'What appears to be the "end" of it all seems so close . . .
It was OK for medieval man with death a mere continuation
of life. For modern man life "ends" before you are dead,
so we have purgatory before annihilation.' Even at the top
of the treadmill there is no hope or real satisfaction.

Your reaction may well be to say that it really isn't as
bad as that. Or perhaps to agree that it might be for many
people, but not for Christians. But if it is different for
Christians, then why do so many succumb to stress, neur-
osis and depression? It is true that humans, like hamsters
and rats, have different genetic make-ups and different
psychological histories which affect considerably the
amount of pressure they can sustain. Some do not succumb
simply because they have stronger physical and psychological constitutions. But what of those who do break under
the strain, the rats like me who fall off exhausted? Is it
simply the inevitable consequence of what we are in
ourselves? Or is it that we are inadequate Christians, defec-
tive in our faith and negligent in our discipline?

We cannot begin to answer these questions until we have
taken a look at the cage and the treadmill, at the many and
converging pressures which are an inevitable part of life in
western society in this last quarter of the twentieth century.
Some pressures are common to both Christian and non-
Christian; others are peculiar to Christians. Those non-
Christian psychiatrists who, in counselling Christians who
have suffered mental breakdown, point the finger at the
church, really have something, since for many Christians
the church commitment is an extra burden and an added
set of real pressures.

It is this situation with which we have to come to terms.
First of all we need to analyse the situation, looking at the
various areas of pressure which form the treadmill on which
our lives are lived. We need to look at the pressures at
work, in social life and in church life which may bring us
to breaking-point.

1
Pressures at work

Professional pressures

Western society worships success. Success is measured in terms of monetary reward, degree of power over others, star quality, professional status, public image, and similar short-lived prizes. Success is not generally evaluated in terms of moral integrity, self-sacrificing compassion, costly adherence to ethical principles, or other biblical standards. Mother Teresa may be admired, but she is rarely copied.

The popularity of *Dallas*, *Dynasty* and kindred programmes reflects this worship. They portray people who have achieved success, financially and in the power game, but whose personal relationships go from crisis to crisis, from disaster to disaster. The tensions and conflicts of the interpersonal relationships actually provide the drama. Without the marriage breakdowns, the ruthless exploitation of others, the transient 'love' relationships and sexual liaisons, the programmes would drop to the bottom of the ratings. Yet all this is accepted as worthwhile – a fair price to pay for achieving the riches and power which, deep down, many yearn for.

The 'macho' image of *Dallas*'s J R may make him a 'baddie', but he is still admired because he makes money, he has power, and he is prepared to use it quite ruthlessly to achieve his own selfish ends. Viewers may secretly hope that J R will get his come-uppance; but if he did the ratings would go down quickly unless some similar outwardly successful but inwardly ruthless character were introduced.

If success in these terms is sought, then it will often be at the cost of personal relationships and by compromising standards and ideals.

C S Lewis, a profound thinker and perceptive observer, pointed out that the basic condition of real success in the political game is to have a ruthless, hard attitude of mind translated into action. Because this attitude in itself generally compromised fundamental Christian virtues, very few fully committed Christians could ever hope to reach the top positions in political life. Probably the last prime minister who consciously tried to be completely guided in all his political life by what he understood to be God's will as a committed Christian, was Gladstone.

The criteria of worldly success are not those of Christian virtue. These criteria are often in direct conflict, producing a constant tension for the committed Christian. Tension means pressure; pressure is an element in stress.

The pressures in some careers are only too clear. In management, the penalty for failure is now not simply lack of promotion, but redundancy. In banking, insurance and other financial organizations, making money is the measure of success, and probably no very searching questions will be asked as to the ethics of the deal. Sailing close to the wind in codes of practice may yield considerable rewards. Tensions arise for the Christian because his perspective of life embraces eternity. That of our present society is largely restricted to achievement in this present life. The reality of death is not faced squarely for it is the end of all hopes and dreams, all possibility of enjoyment and success. The Christian must choose between what he knows he ought to be and what his career is forcing him to be.

The conflict is not new. My paternal grandfather was sacked as a shop manager because he considered that some of the firm's practices should not be engaged in by a Christian, and refused to participate. On the other side of the fence my maternal grandfather resigned from the Co-operative Movement in which he was locally a prominent figure, because he refused to support a cover-up of a fraudulent deal by the local committee, in order to preserve the movement from adverse publicity. There seems to be little evidence that standards of integrity in either industry and commerce or in trade unions and political parties have improved since then; rather the contrary.

Professional pressures come from at least two sources: the *competitive nature* of many careers, and the *moral conflict* between Christian standards and those increasingly accepted as normal, even necessary, in professional and business life.

The world of business does not hold a monopoly in 'professional' pressures. In the academic world of research and teaching, the rat race is also being run. There is the constant compulsion to research and publish before anyone else gets there, to produce the definitive work or the best textbook, and to compromise standards in order to get there first. In addition, the Christian has a moral conflict: how can I, taking my family and church responsibilities seriously, hope to compete successfully with a colleague who spends virtually all his time in the laboratory or the library?

The fiscal policies of the present government have made promotion beyond the lecturer grade in universities so unlikely that the race hardly seems rational if the aim is to get promotion. But such is the nature of fallen man that my belief that I am undoubtedly good enough to beat the rest to the post, however long the odds, is sufficient to push me forward even more ruthlessly. For the Christian the question then becomes even more acute. What – or *who* – am I really working for? And what does my answer to that imply for the race and my participation in it?

Professional groups, especially those in education, are being increasingly drawn into trade union activism. What were once professional associations have become trade unions similar to those of blue collar workers, and Christians who were previously insulated from the peculiar pressures of that area of life are facing the same crises of conscience that some of their brothers have faced for many years. Should a Christian take industrial action? When does a Christian reach the point where he has to go against his union and refuse to submit to its policies?

Monotony

Those in the professions do not generally have to sustain the pressure of sheer monotony. Some things they do are certainly tedious, but routine is punctuated with times of interest, excitement and a real sense of personal achievement. For those in factories, shops and offices – it is another matter. They are part of the 'labour force', a horrid impersonal term which reduces individuals to the level of one pound coins by making them comparable to money. They have to contend with the monotony consequent upon being treated as machines.

Those of us who are 'middle class professionals' too often underestimate the stress caused by such repetitive, inescapable work. The same sequence of actions has to be gone through again and again and again, with no prospect of stopping, however briefly, until the official break. We can act flexibly, they can't. They also face another whole area of stress and pressure. Redundancy and permanent unemployment, already produced by the current economic situation, shadow them. Such 'labour units' are replaced by machines of growing sophistication.

The diary and the timetable

We do, however, let ourselves in for another kind of related pressure – that of the diary and the timetable. The tyranny of these is not confined to secular professionals, for it can apply to ministers of the gospel too, and especially to those who take their work seriously before God. The temptation is to fill every nook and cranny of the day – and night(!) – with some activity or other.

The minister is expected to attend every meeting the church arranges, to look in on the many different organizations and groups with which so many churches are plagued. These are often quite redundant in terms of furthering the kingdom of God. Churches, and probably especially evangelical ones, find it very easy to start an organization or group to meet some specific need. They too often find it impossible to close anything down. The minister finds himself bound to a diary not of his own making, with personal diary commitments to add to the burden. The pressures build as he tries to fit in anything new, and he becomes increasingly conscious that his primary function – the ministry of word and sacrament – begins to suffer. A growing sense of guilt is added to the sheer psychological pressure of rushing from one event to the next.

Active lay Christians also frequently suffer from the constipated diary syndrome. After a full day's work, often with a tight schedule itself, they rush through a meal and off to a meeting at church, or to some para-church organization or mass meeting. They return exhausted to bed, only to wake up to a comparable day's ceaseless activity.

Such a life puts pressure not only on the individual concerned, but also on his family. Most of us have heard of evangelical widows; there are evangelical orphans as well, particularly when children are thought to be old enough to be left at home on their own, or one child is old enough to be made responsible for the rest.

Work schedule

Those in employment are given a work schedule, a set of tasks to be performed, or specific responsibilities to be undertaken. There are important decisions to be taken, meetings with clients or fellow employees, committees, board meetings, lectures, lessons, tutorials, deadlines to be met, targets to be reached, and so on. These are part of our normal pattern of work. They are not bad in themselves. But in two ways they can become so.

First, the time available is crammed with more and more *tasks*. This often happens to the good, conscientious person who can be trusted. Christians, rightly, come into that category. They frequently find themselves asked to do more and more simply because, in a world where standards of honesty, integrity and reliability in any field so often seem to be at a premium, their Christian character makes them obvious candidates for responsibility.

We find it difficult to say, 'No', partly because we feel we ought to say, 'Yes', or simply because we consider it 'bad for the witness' to decline. Perhaps also we feel we shall incur the disapproval of our superiors if we don't take on the work. If we are honest with ourselves, we are flattered by requests to take on more; it shows how much we are needed!

There can also be an element of spiritual pride in it – deep down we feel that we are doing the Lord a bit of good. During my spell serving the king (the secular one!) in the Royal Air Force, a very talented padre told us that he went into the ministry because he felt that the Lord really needed men like him in the full-time service of the church – a motive subsequently repented of with tears.

Dare we admit we fall into the same devilish trap of supposing that we are really quite good chaps (or girls), and the Lord is really rather fortunate to have such talented and responsible and trusted people in his service? May God convict and save us!

The second factor that turns a helpful work schedule into a tyrant is that of *competition*. Many of us are caught up in a highly competitive career structure from which we cannot escape.

It is a catch–22 situation. If we enter the race with the necessary enthusiasm we become subject to almost intolerable stress and pressure if we also try to keep up our Christian zeal and activity to the level we believe we ought. If we opt out and do not treat our job as the number one priority, we feel, rightly or wrongly, that we are discrediting the Lord whom we profess to serve. So we open ourselves to the increasing risk of stress and breakdown.

The more successful we are, the greater the pressures of the race. The higher we climb on the treadmill, the faster the treadmill rotates. It becomes harder and harder to stay where we are. We then either crack under the strain of trying to rise on the treadmill while maintaining our Christian enthusiasm and activity, or (from my observation of generations of Christian students who have moved up in successful careers, this is more likely) the treadmill itself becomes the major preoccupation. Christian faith then becomes simply a matter of maintaining a respectable church attendance, coupled with a money contribution to the work of the church that salves our consciences. We forget 1 Corinthians 3:11–15. As career structure and worldly prospects become paramount, the enthusiastic young Christian becomes the successful, respectable, comfortable, regular churchgoer. In effect, mammon has won. Ultimately the winner becomes the loser.

Failure

Races also have real losers. There are more on the treadmill who make little progress than who succeed. For the ambitious, and perhaps even more for the unambitious man with an ambitious wife, the pressure of failure can be greater than the pressure of success. Despair and depression result, and not uncommonly also a broken marriage – at least in effect, if not publicly demonstrated in separation or divorce.

In a day when failure can so easily mean redundancy and unemployment, the pressures are even greater. Unemployment always produces general despair and loss of identity in anyone who really wants to work, but there is a great deal of evidence which shows that those who have been made redundant from managerial posts go through even greater trauma. Even keen Christians can be broken to tears, full of resentment, bitterness and anger against God, questioning the very faithfulness of the Lord.

Usually the broken come through. My worry is for the man who bottles up his real feelings under a veneer of pious phrases about accepting the Lord's will. It takes a great deal of grace and a truly intimate knowledge of the Lord to say sincerely, 'The Lord gave; the Lord has taken away; blessed be the name of the Lord.' If it is only said because the person thinks it the right thing to say in the company which he keeps then it is only too clear that it is a meaningless cliché. It is also an implicit condemnation of the Christian fellowship in which he feels he has to say it when his whole heart is crying out in anger and resentment. That fellowship can scarcely claim to be showing the compassion of Christ.

Mediocrity

Pressure is not restricted to those who are racing for success or running from failure. It can come from the realization of mediocrity. Coming to terms with the fact that you are not as good as you once thought you were can be hard. It can be even harder if the inevitable disappointment with myself is compounded by the feeling that I have also failed other people – my family, my parents, my children, my teachers, those who have helped me along the way. It is harder still if they, perhaps only by the tone of voice, or the significant look, or, almost unforgivably, the remark overheard or gossiped back, make clear their real feelings on the matter.

Perhaps the pressure of mediocrity is the hardest to bear because it is, almost by definition, most widespread, the least noticed, and the least likely to attract sympathy.

An attempt to expose some of the pressures which relate to working life does not mean that they are all necessarily bad and to be avoided if at all possible. We all need the stimulus of some pressure in order to produce the work for which we were created. Stress and pressure for a period, followed by relaxation and rest, particularly if the activity has been satisfying in itself, produce a sense of achievement. But the short-term achievements gain us nothing lasting if there is no sense of purpose in our life as a whole. Those who are not Christians know, even if they do not admit it, that at the end, however successful they may be, all the pressure and stress will leave them precisely in the same place as the man who has achieved nothing – dead and buried. Christians for whom a living hope in the Lord Jesus is not a practical reality face the same psychological pressure, quite unnecessarily.

2
Pressures in society

Family

Many men, and not a few women, try to combine a demanding career with the responsibilities of family life. Increasingly in our society it has become economically necessary for both husband and wife to work, and this is true for all social groups.

Of course those in higher income groups can afford to employ a nanny, who can very easily become a surrogate mother. Later, the responsibility of parenthood can largely be passed over to the staff of a preparatory school and then a public school. With the growth of independent schools and the increasing wealth of those who are already very well provided for, more families are finding they can do this. Furthermore, there is then increased pressure to achieve success and maintain performance in order to pay for the surrogate parent, so that what is lost on the *family* roundabouts in terms of stress is gained on the *occupational* swings.

What of the ordinary family living together for most of the time? What pressures can be identified there?

My experience is perhaps different from that of most families today. Both our children are now married and each has a child. They were born in Nigeria, and spent the earliest years of their lives in a community of Christians which was very close and caring. During those formative years they escaped many of the pressures which children of Christian parents can suffer when they come up against the different standards and ideals of the world around them.

It is hard enough for the individual parent to be different, it is harder still to demand it of one's children because they belong to a Christian family. Yet if we take the concept of the covenant seriously, as it permeates biblical thought in both testaments, that demand must be made. Perhaps it is hardest of all in the case of teenage children who begin to develop their own individual responsibility and to take decisions for themselves. Such faithfulness to God inevitably creates its own pressures and tensions, and the more so as western society becomes more godless at every level of its life.

There is the constant pressure on parents of the responsibility for their children's well-being. That is readily seen in material terms; but for the Christian there is the additional burden of spiritual responsibility – the prayer, precept and example which children in Christian families need in order to help them grow up into Christ. That involves discipline.

Too often fathers abrogate their responsibilities in that respect and leave it to mothers, a failure which I recognize as I look back on my own experience as a father. Truly loving, Christian discipline is not the legalistic, even sadistic, authoritarianism of so many Victorian fathers. Neither is it the weak reluctance to exercise any authority and punishment to which many fathers so easily succumb in order to avoid conflict. Too often this 'opting out' by fathers places the pressure to discipline solely on the wife.

In modern society, where the successful professional man is so often required to spend periods away from home, the strain and pressure on the wife can become intolerable, particularly where there are two or three children closely spaced. And what if the husband is also active in church work? Even when he *is* home he is *not!* Is it surprising that so many Christian wives live under great pressure, and that the marriage relationship itself comes under severe strain?

Family pressures are by no means restricted to the parents. It is not only adults who succumb to stress and depression. In our society the pressures on children, especially Christian children, are considerable. There are children even in primary school who have endured active, even vicious, persecution simply because they come from Christian families, and are prepared to say so – and be proud of it. Then, as they grow up, the pressures on children increase. During school years there is examination competition and the pressure to achieve, and at the end the constant fear of unemployment.

How many parents *add* to the pressure by looking for vicarious satisfaction out of the success of their children? Many parents do not realize the subtle pressures they apply in this area, even if they do not *actively* press their children to achieve, either at school or in other areas of life. If Christian parents were honest with themselves or, more importantly, with God, how many would have to admit that it is more important to them that their children succeed – in the worldly sense – than that they should come to know and love and serve the Lord, *even at the cost of* worldly success?

Pressure by parents is not restricted to young children. The hold that some try to retain over their married offspring is quite frightening, and not only in situations where one parent has died and the other thus left alone. In such a situation it is understandable, if not excusable, that the surviving parent should have expectations of the married children. It is right that married children should take a share of responsibility for a bereaved parent. There are many cases where the expectations are, however, quite wrong and unhealthy. The children and their spouses are expected to be on call for quite trivial errands, or to make a weekly, and often much more frequent, visit, and to treat it as *the* priority. Sometimes the visit of the parents to the children implicitly takes the form of an inspection of domestic arrangements and is often highly critical. The criticism takes the form of mother (or mother-in-law) setting to on a cleaning session, or father (or father-in-law) engaging in an unsought do-it-yourself job.

When will parents take seriously the implications of the verse: 'a man will *leave his father and mother* and be united to his wife'? There are two sides to marriage: the intimate relation between husband and wife, which becomes the primary relationship; and the leaving of parents, which means that they must take the complementary step of giving up their child to his wife or to her husband. This is hard; I know because I have had to do it. It takes real self-discipline and self-denial; but it leads to a far richer relationship than does the attempt to maintain some form of relationship akin to the pre-adult link. Sometimes, unfortunately, it is the children who have to force the break in order to preserve and develop their marriage relationship.

To quote the effective working of the extended family in many societies is no answer to this point. In such societies the roles of the various members of the family are well-defined, recognized and observed. In our society such a framework has broken down and has not been replaced by another appropriate to the nuclear family which characterizes our social system.

Marriage

The basic marriage relationship is also under strain, even among Christians – good evangelical Christians. In our secular society it is now almost assumed that a marriage relationship will not last. The prevailing view is that it can't be expected to because we fall in and out of love so easily, and success in marriage is supposed to depend upon how we feel. The ideological pressure on the stability of marriage is considerable because the attitude of society totally contradicts the biblical view.

The whole situation becomes an intensified complex of pressures when it is coupled with the demands made by the professional lifestyle typical of so many today. Success in a career now depends on how willing a person is to be mobile, to spend frequent or long periods away from home on business, or at conferences and seminars. Marital tension is thus coupled with both temptation and opportunity, in an atmosphere in which unfaithfulness is almost a norm, or at best a mere triviality. With more couples seeking to combine a career for each with marriage and family life, the slide into sin is open to both partners.

Adultery is not a new sin; it is now just easier to commit. Victorian men did it in secret; contemporary men and women do it openly. This is no exaggeration, even in Christian families. There are many broken marriages involving Christians, and many more which have come close to breakdown. Even clergy marriages break down – and so commonly that they no longer make the *News of the World*, unless they are accompanied by particularly lurid circumstances.

Security for the future

This is another pressure on the family. We see our future security in terms of financial provision. In a monetary economy prudence dictates that we must. The welfare state had in some ways begun to alleviate such concern; but can we any longer rely on that? Anyway, most people in industry and the professions wish to go beyond the provision of the state and to try to insure for every conceivable eventuality. Further, the advertisements in the press and the invitations through the mail never allow us to get away from the pressure to invest more and more of our present resources to provide for a 'secure' future.

I have no wish to devalue prudence, indeed our Lord commended it; but he also warned against the dangers of laying up treasure on earth at the expense of treasure in heaven. Perhaps some of us come very near to relying more on our pension funds and life insurance policies for our future security, than upon an omnipotent God who loves us. Our Lord promised that, if we put him and his affairs first, everything else would be added as a bonus, though he doesn't promise to provide all we *want*, only what we *need*. The two standards may be very different, since the first is highly conditioned by our expectations, which are dependent to a great degree upon the presuppositions of our culture, society and social group. Those expectations need to be examined in the light of God's word.

We profess to serve a Lord who said to one who would follow him that his creatures had nests and lairs, but he had nowhere to lay his head. The crucial question is where our *real* trust lies in relation to the future. I fear that for many evangelical Christians security in this life is based upon adequate insurance, and that the salvation which we say we have through faith in Jesus Christ is in practice little more than the ultimate life insurance policy to take care of us when the other insurances can no longer provide the necessary cover.

Social conscience

There is, however, an opposite pressure. Those of us who are relatively well-heeled cannot be ignorant of the plight of the majority of our fellow human beings. Most of them live in dire poverty, in stark contrast to our comfort and wealth. If we are at all sensitive our consciences will be stirred. Though we may give generously to relief agencies, we are still not satisfied that such gifts are enough, because we know that we are part of the structures which maintain and contribute to such poverty and deprivation. We are also naggingly aware that we can do nothing to change them. To Spirit-sensitized souls the pressure can be subtle and persistent – a burden that cannot be shed.

As I reflect on my own breakdown, I am more than ever convinced that my living and travelling in many parts of Africa was a constant rub on a raw nerve. My wider travels since then still produce a deep and elusive pain, which is constantly reactivated by the news items which occupy our television screens and newspapers.

Our social conscience has a wider significance. Kenneth Leech, in his book *The Social God* (Sheldon, 1981), has argued that the Christian faith will only be able to speak prophetically to society if it has a vision for where that society should be going. Without the vision the church's voice is hollow and pointless, but the true vision, sought and obtained in the quietness of worship, contemplation and communion with the living God must inevitably lead to a prophetic voice which demands articulation.

The closer we are to God in our worship and personal devotion, the more grieved and hurt we shall be by the deep evil, injustice, intolerance, selfishness, hatred, bigotry, arrogance and blatant cruelty which are to be found in all societies, of whatever political complexion.

The more sensitive we become the more impotent we shall feel. Followers of Christ cannot salve their consciences or ease the tension by shifting the blame on to particular groups or political parties. The closer we are to the Lord, the more sensitive we shall be and the deeper will be our agonizing over the evil in ourselves and the evil which permeates all the structures of society. This is not to devalue in any way the kindness, goodness and concern which can be found by the common grace of God amidst the evil; we thank God for it. But we can still see that evil permeates the whole.

Consider, for example, this typical political or industrial

situation. One side accuses the other of some serious misdemeanour. This is strongly denied by the side accused. If it is found that they really are in the wrong, they have added dishonesty to it. If the accusation turns out to be false, the accusers are shown to be liars. Even if the lie is based on false information received sincerely as true, guilt merely lies one step further back with those who fabricated the accusation. The Christian ought to be sensitive to such facts of life in our society. Christians active in politics or industrial relations in any capacity must be especially conscious of such stresses and pressures; but they ought not to be alone, for we all ought to be socially sensitive. However, it must be recognized that this constitutes yet another subtle pressure.

Secularism

Another form of pressure underlies a number of areas we have already looked at. It is the simple fact that we as Christians live in a pagan society.

Modern western man is content to accept the life of the cage. Secularization has now reached the point where there are hardly any signs left of Christian attitudes and values. Relativistic morals – personal, social and political – now hold the field. Crucial ethical issues, such as experimentation on human embryos, abortion and euthanasia are thought through and evaluated purely in terms of the ethical assumptions accepted within the cage.

A very plausible and moving argument often advanced for experimentation on human embryos is that it will enable us to understand genetic disorders which produce handicapped babies. This will enable us to eliminate, for example, haemophilia; so such scientific advances will remove some of the causes of family and personal unhappiness and hardship. Since we assume that the human embryo cannot, in any meaningful sense, experience happiness or pain, the balance of happiness is clearly weighted in favour of the fully developed human being, born and independent. Here it is not my purpose to criticize this argument in itself, but merely to point out that it is based solely upon a utilitarian assumption that an act which promotes the happiness of the greatest number is in itself good. The Christian will want to introduce other arguments into the discussion which are not utilitarian, but prescriptive and related to the revelation of God in Jesus Christ. In most debates today those arguments will be seen as irrelevant to practical action, and dismissed as the consequence of religious 'fanaticism'.

Whether or not the Christian has thought through his position on such matters, his general background of teaching will produce a subconscious tension between his own instinctive position and that which he senses in the arguments of those who do not share his ethical presuppositions. If he is articulate on such matters, he will lay himself open to snide remarks about being 'Victorian', 'Fundamentalist' or even 'unchristian'. Such jibes reveal more about the ignorance of those who make them than about the views of those referred to; but they still hurt. They point up the essential tension which is constantly present between the Christian and the world in which he lives.

We commonly speak of that world as being 'secular', and of the 'increasing secularization' of western society. The *truly* secular man is a rarity – the man for whom all religious categories are completely irrelevant or obsolete. Probably he exists principally in universities, and then only among certain highly-disciplined intellectuals. His students, however, are likely to be into astrology, the occult, drugs or transcendental meditation. Organized religion is certainly on the decline overall, though even this must be qualified by the fact that many local churches are growing.

Science may also be seen as having debunked Christianity as a credible revelation. But the intellectual assertion that there is nothing outside the material world has not killed the desire that there should be. It seems to be inherent in man. What has happened is that religion has become 'privatized', as Kenneth Leech so aptly puts it. That is, religion is seen as a purely personal matter; it satisfies an individual yearning which will not go away. As such it poses no threat to social systems, and asks no questions about social morality; it succeeds in divorcing totally the spiritual dimension from the material life of man. This is not confined to the many false beliefs and practices which abound in a culture where 'anything goes' so long as it anaesthetizes the religious pain in the human psyche. The privatization of religion is apparent in much that professes to be Christian, even evangelically Christian. The emphasis is so often upon *personal* morality, *personal* salvation, *individual* experience, *private* peace and satisfaction. All of these are important, but deficient – and dangerously so – in two ways.

First, an introspective, partial vision is just as idolatrous as a false vision; in biblical terms it *is* a false vision and can lead to the most dangerous idolatry of all – a growing cancer of self-preoccupation.

Second, it opens the way to the insidious growth of spiritual schizophrenia. All of us are in part products of our cultural environment; it is part of us. For the vast majority of our lives we participate in the ongoing life of that culture as it is expressed in the society in which we live. If our faith has nothing worthwhile to say about our relation to that society and, more importantly, about God's relation to it, then we are deprived of the spiritual equipment to cope with a major part of our lives. That part becomes progressively divorced from the 'spiritual' bit, and the psychological pressure becomes more and more intense. We need to see how our daily, 'secular' work can be just as much God's service as, for instance, leading the young people's fellowship at church.

Many of us have social obligations which are part and parcel of the job we do – the responsibility to entertain guests or engage in other activities – and we have to decide how far along these roads we ought to go, if we go at all. Unless we are content with a narrow and arbitrary legalism, which is the easy way out, we need to know what God's relation to our work is, and what he requires of us in it. That cannot be answered in purely personal and individual terms since its reference is much wider. What would your answer be to the question, 'What role does your job have in your Christian life?' Or to, 'What vision do you have for your career in God's purpose for this world?' I suggest that, 'As a place for Christian witness' is an inadequate answer to the first; and that, 'As a means of providing me with the necessary money to live so that I can work for Christ in my spare time' is just as inadequate in the case of the second. Both answers imply a tension between serving God, and serving the boss or 'myself'. The tension is a source of pressure, and needs to be resolved.

3
Pressures in the church

Servicing activities

Surely when we turn to the local Christian community to which we belong we should expect to find a release from stress and pressure? Maybe we should, but far too often it is not the case. We simply encounter another complex of pressures.

Instead of being worshipping bodies in the unity of the Spirit, local churches are too often mere meeting places for restricted-interest groups each doing its own thing – no doubt a holy or an evangelistic or a spiritual thing, but still its *own*. All these groups rarely come together. Even the Sunday morning congregation has few members in common with that of Sunday evening. Children may be present for part of the morning service, and even for the whole when we have a family service, but what sighs of relief there are when the children are led out and the adults can then get down to the real business of undistracted worship – that is, to *doing their own thing*. Weekly *family* services can too easily become *children's* services, without sufficient meat to bring adults to growth. Some adults deliberately don't come. Instead, they'll go to the evening worship.

How often do church members complain that individuals never get to know one another? What else can we expect if the whole organization is geared to the needs of a hundred-and-one separate groups, each with its own interests and its own distinctive membership? The reasons for this are not far to seek.

First, most churches find it *easy to start activities*, but find it almost *impossible to close any down*.

Take the example of Sunday school. The movement started as a way of instructing the illiterate children of the poor in basic skills like reading and writing. The vehicle for teaching was the Christian faith through the Bible. It then became a general activity for the instruction of all the children in the church. With the advent of universal primary education the original purpose was redundant, but the Sunday school continued as an essential element in church activity, providing Christian teaching for children, including those of church members. It took place in the afternoon so that such children came to morning worship as well, as part of the family, and often in the evening also. Then, with the increasing mobility provided by the motor car, and the attraction of television, Sunday sport and entertainment, Sunday afternoon attendances fell, even from church families.

Then Sunday school became 'Children's church' and coincided with morning worship, thus depriving children of the experience of the worship of the body of Christ in its fullness. Now we try to mix the two, and we have 'Family Worship'. It is often so geared to the children that the adults are deprived of real spiritual food unless they are prepared to come in the evening, which all too few are disposed to do. This is not a criticism of Sunday school or Family Worship as such; the question is whether there may not be better ways of providing appropriate instruction for both children and adults, while preserving the full unity of the local congregation.

We need to think radically and more fundamentally about the whole question. At the moment we are hamstrung by history, and multiply divisions on the basis of age. It is no wonder that teenagers fail to take to adult worship when the time comes. We nurture them with the idea that age is the supreme division in the local church; we encourage them to think that they are different, and that the next step, into full worship, is optional.

Some churches, as an accountant friend of mine put it, seem to be little more than holding companies for a large number of essentially separate businesses engaged in a multitude of different activities. Tragically many of those activities are already bankrupt and beyond being bailed out by the diminishing resources of the holding company. The pressure on the leaders is therefore much the same as that on businessmen in a similar predicament.

Keeping the activities going then becomes more important than prayer and worship, which are treated as though they were activities among other activities, of similar value and equally optional. The local church thus denies its essential life, and deprives those who work in the organizations of the spiritual resourses they need in order to work to real spiritual effect.

Churches need to engage in periodic pruning to get rid of excess branches which no longer bear fruit. Every local congregation would do well to prune back to the base stock every five years. That stock is *worship*, through the ministry of word and sacrament and corporate praise and intercessory prayer. Only those activities which are demonstrably bearing fruit to God's glory would be grafted back on to the stock. This would be hard because the hold of history is difficult to break, and there are often vested interests at work to keep particular groups going. For those individuals who belong to them, that group *is* the church. In God's sight it is not.

Second, *many churches have lost the vision of the centrality of worship*. Public acts of worship and meeting for corporate prayer are seen simply as particular activities among many, of at least equal importance, in which the church is engaged. In fact they are the foundation activities of the whole church without which the rest are worthless, and might just as well disappear.

The church is at root a spiritual body deriving its life and nourishment from God alone. Cut that out or weaken it and, though it may have form, it has little or no real spiritual life however active it may appear to be in terms of the organizations and groups listed on its notice-board and in its monthly magazine. That life, and the vision which is necessary for all its other activities, is derived *only* from the worship and prayer of the whole body of Christians who make up the congregation.

We need to recover the New Testament vision of the church as something more than a collection of committed individuals, and of membership in the church as being a living organ in a vital, vibrant body, whose corporate life is as vital as the lives of its individual members. Until we do, we shall continue to expend tremendous energy to little purpose, with all the pressure and stress that is included for those who have to maintain the activities.

The ultimate solution to the problem is to recover the priorities of the New Testament which are set out in Acts 2:42–47. What that might mean in practice would require another book to work out fully. It is important, however, to draw attention to the fact that pressures in the church situation are not inevitable and unavoidable. They are certainly not an essential part of serving Christ in his church. They are largely a consequence of past events and developments over which we have no control. But it is in our control to hand on to the next generation a situation that is healthier than the one we have inherited.

Para-church groups

The nineteenth and twentieth centuries have seen a huge growth in extra- and para-church organizations. Some of them fulfil important functions in the economy of God. They all have to be staffed and serviced, often by the same people who are in demand by the local church. Moreover, if the local church is in effect a rag-bag of disparate organizations and groups, where do those who work in important para-church organizations find their real spiritual roots and the church support in prayer and worship on which their effectiveness depends? The conflict of loyalties that can result provides another source of stress and pressure, without the reservoir of spiritual strength to cope with it provided in the prayer and worship of the body of Christ.

Misunderstandings between groups

Whether he recognizes it or not, the church worker's desire to make his own group activity a success will also be a factor in promoting stress. Inter-group rivalry is not unknown in churches! When the roles of organizations in the church overlap rivalry can be particularly acute.

For example, the minister's wife sometimes finds herself at the centre of a group of warring women's groups. Youth groups and music groups may also be culprits. Of course, they do not actually fight; they merely do one another down verbally, and every titbit of gossip is used as ammunition in the battle.

The letters in the New Testament have a great deal to say about the way God sees gossip, innuendo, and evil-speaking – more than about many other sins of which we are far more conscious and censorious. The more groups there are, the more likely it is that misunderstandings and tensions will arise.

Differences in doctrinal emphasis

Then there are the groups which arise in congregations over differences of doctrinal emphasis – for example, the divisions produced by the view of the more spectacular gifts of the Spirit, like tongues and healings; or between the 'Reformed' and the 'less Reformed'; or between radical evangelicals and those with a more pietistic streak; or concerning the acceptability or not of rock gospel music.

Such differences are probably inevitable when scripture itself is so rich and its truth cannot be captured completely within any one set of pigeonholes devised by men. But it is wrong when one group either openly or by implication treats another as inferior in God's sight because of the views they hold. We must certainly contend for the truth – but in Christlike love, remembering that the answer to error is not to be found primarily in its intellectual refutation, but rather by the demonstration of the truth in both the way we live and the way we speak. *There* is another source of tension and stress.

Within the church, his infernal majesty (to use C S Lewis's phrase) is a master of exploiting all such differences to the full in order to make the work of God ineffective. How easy it is for God's people to cooperate with him in his insidious undermining of what the Lord wants to achieve through his church!

Lack of corporate life

All church activities should grow out of corporate prayer and corporate worship, and should only be maintained as long as they continue to flow out from this vital centre of church life. If this is not happening there will be two results.

First, much effort will be expended on activities which will do little to build up Christ's church. This is because they will lack the dynamic which is the essence of true spiritual success – the power of the Spirit of God, directing and working.

Second, those who are committed to working in these activities will be denied the only real source of strength for coping with the pressures those activities bring. Just knowing that the whole church is supporting with prayer the work one does in the church can be a tremendous strength, comfort, and release in the pressure which is inherent in any spiritual battle.

All real work for the Lord is part of the ultimate battle between God and the forces of cosmic evil. Paul often refers to this in his letters to the churches which were so dear to him (see, for example, Rom 8:37–39; Eph 3:7–11; 6:10–12; Col 2:15). That is a pressure which inevitably faces all who would truly serve the Lord. The answer to it is to be found in the working out in our daily lives of the victory of Christ over that enemy. To do that is hard, but it will be even harder if we try to do it without the overt support of our fellow members in the body of Christ. We need to draw corporately on Christ's strength and the power of his victory.

The imagery of the Christian's armour – which we are exhorted to put on *with prayer* – is drawn from the equipment of the Roman soldier. Despite his armour, he would have been useless if he had to fight the battle alone. His strength lay in the fact that he was part of a highly-disciplined, fully organized and strictly trained legion in the army of Rome. The implications of Paul's image are clear.

So, then, who is it who trains, organizes and disciplines the army of the living God? Christ, the head of the church, by his Spirit. That training, disposition and discipline take place in the corporate worship and prayer of the church of Christ.

Conformity

There are legitimate pressures in the service of God; but many other pressures to which those who would serve the Lord are subject are brought about by the imperfections of the churches and situations in which we work. Some of these are hard to avoid, but all of them would be reduced if we began to get our priorities right in the local church.

For example, there is the pressure to conform. Local churches have established patterns of doing things, both in worship and other activities. Such patterns become fixed and deviations are not tolerated, often for no better reason than, 'We have always done it this way here.'

This sort of response is very frustrating for active newcomers and for young people coming to maturity in Christ with the ideas of a new generation. If it is a constant, repeated experience then it becomes stressful, a significant pressure on them. It is particularly harmful for the person who has a strong streak of loyalty to his church – in other words for the person who is likely to be of most real value to that church.

It is hardly surprising that the house church movement seems to have become such a haven for disaffected members of the established denominations; too many churches almost seem to go out of their way to produce disaffected members. The house church movement, however, seems to have its own problems as a result of imposing a conformity of a rather different kind on its members.

It is not only young Christians who face this pressure. A new minister, going into an old-established and strongly-led congregation, may see much that needs changing. He has a vision of where the church should be going, but at every point he is frustrated by his Parochial Church Council, his Kirk Session, his elders, his deacons, or his church committee.

Demands of demanding people

The minister has many demands made upon him by his congregation or parish. The demands come from a wide range of different groups, with different needs and widely varying expectations of what the minister should do.

A group of Anglican ordinands I was with spent a week of their training looking at the problems of both urban and rural ministry. One task was to think about the expectations that people in the parish might have of the parish clergy – even though those people might not be very committed to corporate worship. We put these probable expectations in order of priority. We did the same for those who were devoted to worship and the spiritual dimensions of church life, and found that the priorities were almost completely reversed.

With limited time, and his own view of what his priorities should be, the church minister is obviously going to suffer the tensions of many conflicting expectations.

Such pressures exist to some degree for all who would bear spiritual responsibility in the church of Christ. In addition to deciding priorities, people with problems – real or imagined – make a considerable demand on the leader's emotions as well as his time. The imaginary problems often create the most stress, both for the counsellor and the counselled. Imaginary problems arise from our inability to face up to ourselves as we really are, and to get rid of our delusions, whether of grandeur or inferiority. Imaginary problems can, however, produce *real* stress and *real*, observable symptoms.

The leader's family

Added to all these pressures which seem to focus on ministers and leaders, there is considerable resultant stress and pressure on their wives and families.

When the minister is out on one of his many calls, whether to individuals or to groups engaged in activities associated with the church, who is it who takes the phone calls, bears the obvious displeasure of those who find that the minister is not at their immediate call, takes the messages, listens to those who will not ring off? The minister's wife! And so often those who call do not stop to consider the leader's family, calling at meal-times, bed-times, and other times of special domestic activity.

On balance, how many of the calls which come at critical times in family life are really all that urgent? Church leaders are entitled to expect something better of the members of their flocks, who at least profess to be Christians. Many clergy find it very difficult to say, 'No, I'm sorry, it can't be done now; I'll come round tomorrow (or next week, or as soon as I can make it).'

Of course there are urgent needs that have to be met, there are calls which require immediate attention; but there are also many which do not, but for which immediate attention is *demanded*. The experience of many ministers and leaders is that it is usually those in deepest need who are most considerate towards the one attempting to meet the need.

The minister is not an amateur social worker; nor is he the managing director of a company with many functions and activities. He is a minister of word and sacrament – even if the sacraments are called ordinances! That is the function to which he has been called by God, trained to perform, and set apart by the church of Christ to fulfil.

Having been a layman in the church for thirty-five or more active years before I was ordained, I have seen the situation from *both* sides. Perhaps, because of that, I am more able to cope now that I am ordained than many of my younger friends who have less experience of being a layman – and are also having to cope with the additional responsibility, now no longer mine, of having a growing family at home.

Expectations of holiness

Of course, the minister or church worker caught in this ceaseless round of activity is expected not to suffer under the strain. After all *he* has access to unique supernatural grace and a power of the Spirit which should carry him serenely through all the pressures which work, family and church bring to bear upon him! If he complains or succumbs, there is clearly something wrong with his faith. If there are tensions at home, in his family and marriage, then he or she will feel bound to hide them because it is 'so bad for the witness' when these things get out. Such unrealistic expectations only reinforce the minister's stress and tension.

Guilt feelings

Two things result from trying to maintain a large number of church organizations and activities. First, churches are under constant pressure to keep them all staffed. And, second, the willing are pressed into more and more responsibility.

The pressure of these excessive demands then turns into a deep sense of guilt at not being able to meet them all adequately. The expectations of anyone with vision will gradually seem more and more remote from what is actually being achieved, and the possibility of getting any closer seems increasingly unlikely. Frustration increases, the joy of service disappears, and the sense of abject failure begins to sour the church worker's relationship with God. This fosters a subconscious sense of guilt which festers deep in the personality.

The tragedy is that the real guilt is not that of the person who breaks down under the strain, but that of the church which imposes in this way on the willing, devoted Christian servant. It is not that any individual is, necessarily, to blame. Rather it is the structure, which generations have unthinkingly allowed to develop, that produces the stress, increases the pressure, and causes the guilt. It is the structure itself – now accepted as the norm – which breaks those people who are involved in keeping it going.

Technique

Modern technological society has made its own distinctive contribution to this creaking superstructure. Instead of a radical examination of the foundations and the building, we seek our salvation in techniques – in relation to youth work, to evangelism, to church growth, and even in prayer and Bible study. The perceived priority for the church worker is that he or she should be technically competent. Spiritual maturity is all too often a secondary qualification. So there is the pressure to attend courses, to acquire techniques, to become an efficient performer in the assigned role.

Technical competence is not to be despised. On the contrary, the individual who works for God has a real responsibility to develop his gifts and become master of the role he is called to play in the church. Nor are techniques in teaching, in music, in youth work or in Bible study to be underrated. But what is quite wrong is the unspoken assumption that if the right technique is developed then all will be well . . . *If only* the right programme for church growth is employed then declining numbers will be changed into an increasing congregation. *If only* the right techniques are applied to the work with our young people then they will be converted and flock to worship. *If only* the right pattern of worship is developed then our dull liturgies – both Anglican and nonconformist – will suddenly spring to attractive and fulfilling life. *If only* modern musical idioms are used, then a vital, new expression of spiritual experience will ensure living worship.

A case could be made out that the emphasis on techniques

is the major idolatry of the church today. If we examine our churches honestly is it not true that too often we rely on techniques rather than on God working by his Spirit? This puts further pressure on time and effort, and we should ask whether it is time rightly spent in terms of spiritual goals. It is inevitable that time spent in the acquisition of technical expertise can often only be bought at the expense of time which should be spent in spiritual preparation, so that again we meet the conflict between the time spent doing, and that spent being and growing. The latter is the only real route to *doing* effectively without unbearable stress and strain.

I am not saying that technique is unimportant, or that change, modern idioms in worship, new teaching methods or other aids are unnecessary. I *am* asserting that the spiritual maturity of those engaged in church work is primary. This maturity can come *only* by the work of the Holy Spirit through worship including both the ministry of the word and the sacraments, and corporate as well as private devotion and intercession. Everything else follows from that and depends on it. Reliance, whether explicit or implicit, upon technical competence, however sound and valid, is nothing short of idolatry. In the end it will do little good and perhaps much harm in the church of Christ. The harm is beginning to be seen in the number of devoted, sincere and spiritual Christian workers who come to breaking-point.

The church of Christ in its local expression has too often become simply a second mill which Christians have to tread in addition to the secular treadmill of their daily lives. Much taxing activity that has no real impact seems to be the picture in a disturbing number of churches. It appears that the church succeeds in breaking a significant number of its full-time workers, including clergy. If *that* is the case, what chance does the dedicated lay worker have when there are *two* treadmills available to run on?

4
Stop the mill;
I want to get off!

Perhaps what has been written so far has rung the occasional bell in your mind. If it has struck a whole ring of changes, then begin to be concerned and be prepared for a radical reappraisal of your whole life. To neglect to undertake an honest examination and to act on its findings will result in a re-examination being forced on you by your arrival at the breaking-point.

How can we go about self-examination and the consequent reordering of our lives? That will depend upon the theological perspective we adopt. It is the cage which creates the need for the treadmill, and the cage represents the view which we take of the world. Only if it is possible to break out of the cage can the treadmills be straightened out and turned into ladders.

The happy pagan runs on one treadmill; when the church is seduced into reducing her vision to the inside of the cage then inevitably her activities become a treadmill too. It is only by the recovery of the perspective from the outside of the cage that both treadmills can be turned into a single ladder, which is what is needed. That is a theological task to which we turn in the next major section of the book.

Unavoidable pressure

There are, however, some relevant comments to be made at this point. First, *some pressure and stress in life is unavoidable, and may not be a bad thing*. Competition can be a stimulus to effort and achievement of which we never dreamt we were capable. Effort and pressure, however, need to be followed by effective relaxation. The problem today is that it is difficult to get the balance, especially for the Christian, who may well be running on two treadmills and who, in our pagan and idolatrous society, is subject to stresses the happy pagan knows nothing of.

Second, *it is the convergence of presssures on the individual which constitutes the crux of the problem*. Single areas of pressure and stress, for example, in a marriage, can and do produce individual breakdown, but generally the danger is most apparent when pressures in two or more areas of life converge. Then the danger is real.

In my own case there was the pressure of illness, and the stress of teenage children at home; there was deep frustration with what seemed to me to be the shortsighted policies of a new head of department who was out of sympathy with my own radical ideas of the changes needed; at church there was a vacancy which produced divisions concerning the kind of minister we needed, and there was the beginning of the debates associated with the formation of the United Reformed Church.

I saw myself as the perfect – or at least rather good – father at home; as the only member of the department with any real vision and ideas at the university; and as a latter-day Luther at church.

Each perception was a lie of the devil. There wasn't time to think things through, nor did I think it necessary. I was caught in my own web of frustration which bound me to the treadmills of my life. I could not break free, but tragically I do not think I ever saw the necessity to break free.

I was utterly convinced that I was doing the will of the Lord, and that the pressure and stress were the unavoidable corollary of following that will. As I saw it, to give up anything would be to concede defeat on matters of vital principle, and that would have been a tragedy not to be countenanced. The bitter irony was that in the end I was defeated in every area in which I was under pressure. Nothing changed at the university, nor was anything achieved at church. Had I been prepared to retreat strategically and graciously in one or the other, or perhaps in both, the domestic pressures and my response to them would have been very different. It is sad that when Christians are under pressure at work and in church it is family life – the area which should be preserved most jealously – which often suffers.

Third, the problem is not simply the convergence of pressures but that, viewed from within the network of differing stresses and strains, *the whole complex seems inevitable*. The victim ties himself to his treadmills. He often does not even see the need to detach himself from any of them. 'Defeat' is unthinkable and so, like a neurotic rat, he runs ever more frantically until he falls off exhausted.

Opting out?

The attractive option which immediately suggests itself is to retreat out of society, the organized church and the work environment, to a secluded commune of like-minded Christians. Surely there one could find freedom from pressure and stress in a wholly Christian environment –

something of a modern equivalent to the medieval closed monastic order. Unfortunately, in some such communities the vow of chastity may prove necessary in order to combat adultery; poverty serves to exacerbate the tensions; and true charisma is debased into a devilish psychological dominance.

Some communities have, of course, proved successful, but generally *their* vision has *not been escapist*, but rather to witness to a different form of Christian lifestyle. Even then, an escape from pressure and stress may not be found but rather a change from one set of pressures to a different set.

There are valid arguments for establishing a visible, alternative Christian lifestyle as a witness to the social implications of the Christian gospel. There is on the other hand no biblical support for the view that all Christians are called to take that route, or that it is in some way more holy. That would be to repeat the error of medievalism. The monastic calling was seen as higher than the secular vocation, so many for whom it was not a true vocation entered it with lasting damage to the cause of Christ.

Since jumping off the treadmill and forming our own small nest in the corner of the cage is probably not a real option for the majority of us, the only other option for the Christian is, by God's grace, to turn the treadmill into a ladder. Unfortunately, too many of us begin to think of that too late, after succumbing to the many stresses and pressures which converge on us. Too often, when we do break under the strain, the same church or congregation that increased our load of pressure shows a singular and culpable lack of understanding, sympathy and practical help; all things which might contribute significantly to our recovery. We are treated as spiritual failures, defeated Christians, weak fainthearts who mar the witness of the church to Christ.

Breaking point

The pressure accumulates. It all focuses on me. As it grows, my psychological and physiological constitution becomes increasingly stretched; but I may well be quite unaware that the tension is having any effect. Then, suddenly, my constitution can stand it no longer. In protest it musters its own defences and reacts, so that I *cannot* continue. Severe clinical depression sets in, accompanied by stress reactions in the cardio-vascular system or by other physiological symptoms of neurotic origin – even complete nervous breakdown or a heart attack. My overstressed systems have broken down. My increased sensitivity to stress and pressure may also express itself in allergic reactions of one kind or another.

It is important to realize that though the symptoms are neurotic in origin they are not therefore imaginary; they are real, measurable, identifiable, sensible symptoms.

The popular view in Christian congregations, especially in the case of clinical depression, is that the *symptoms* are 'all in the mind', and all that the patient needs to do is to pull himself together, to exercise faith, to deepen trust, to pray for healing, and all will be well. Failure to recover is seen as evidence of a defeated Christian. The final defeat is for the treatment to involve being either an out- or an in-patient at the local psychiatric unit. Drugs are suspect and indicators · of third-rate Christianity; electro-convulsive therapy (when wisely used, often a successful – but not clearly understood – treatment for clinical depression) is the sign of irrevocable defeat.

Many, perhaps most, Christians find it much easier to cope with physical than mental illness, and physical handicap than mental handicap. This is reflected in our attitudes to the individuals who suffer from them. We may try very hard to hide our deep, almost subconscious, discrimination; but it certainly is detected by the sufferer to whom we try to present a rather different image.

I have not only been blessed – and I mean that – by

experiencing deep depression and severe physiological symptoms of intolerable stress; I have also been blessed with a mentally handicapped sister. I found it very difficult to come to terms with that fact, but over the years my whole appreciation of such handicaps has been transformed; and not without pain. I have been challenged at the deepest level concerning the reality of my own professed *agape*. I have also seen what the grace of God has done in my sister's life in bringing her to a reality of faith and absolute trust in the Lord Jesus which shames mine. This has made me realize that my judgments do not match the Lord's – though they ought to! Truly God has chosen the weak of this world to confound the wise.

Those who are brought low by physical and mental breakdown *can* rise to new heights of service and reach deeper levels of trust through their affliction, even if they have, quite literally, brought it on themselves. The rats who fall off can build a new ladder to glory. No one can fall so low that he cannot be raised again to new levels of active service for the Lord, to experience a more profound faith, and to come to a deeper knowledge of God than was even imagined before the breaking-point.

How can that be? How can the breaking-point be avoided? Is it in fact necessary to come to that point before such deeper experiences of the Lord may be known? Such questions must now be examined.

PART TWO

The view
from outside the cage:

how God sees our activity

5
Blindness in the cage

The spectacle of rats in a cage, frantically and fruitlessly running on a treadmill, makes a tragic comedy. Their competitive jostling for position is amusing, but the tragedy of their situation also strikes us. 'Poor things!' we say, 'how tragic to be confined like that, spending so much energy getting nowhere.' The situation is even more tragic if there is, close to the treadmill, a ladder leading out of the top of the cage into full freedom. But the motion of the treadmill holds a strange fascination for the rats, and few attempt the ladder. Yet a ladder is only a straightened-out treadmill. The rats seem blind to the way of escape – providing the same kind of exercise, but actually getting somewhere.

The tragedy is even greater when *Christian* rats become fascinated by the hypnotic motion of the treadmill. On

Sundays, and perhaps occasionally in the week, they take a quick jump over to the ladder, climb a few rungs, and then go back to the treadmill. Then back to the ladder, in effect to climb the same few rungs again; perhaps a few more than last week, perhaps a few less, but never making real and permanent progress.

Could that be how God sees the cage of our limited horizons and the treadmill which we have made of daily living?

Ignoring God in practical living

It is easy to think of those in our churches and circle of friends to whom the picture applies. I did in the early 1970s – but, of course, it didn't apply to me!

I could cope. I was 100% for the Lord in everything. I only wanted his way and his will. But I *was* rather peeved that I didn't get a senior lectureship when I thought I had earned one, and I *was* offended when others were asked to contribute to seminars and I wasn't.

Many other things were also symptoms of the fact that I was on the treadmill of self-effort rather than the ladder of discipleship during the week and, as a consequence, my attempts to ascend the ladder when I leapt on to it in worship and church activity became even more frantic – a sure prescription for reaching breaking-point pretty quickly. I received a deserved rebuke from an older Christian minister – 'Get this into your head! If the Lord wants you to have a senior lectureship, you will get it; if he doesn't, then there is nothing on earth that you can do to get one. So go and get on with the work he has given you to do.' Even this, though making a tremendous impact on me intellectually, did not work its way into the fibre of my Christian living until after the Lord had allowed me to come to breaking-point.

The subtlety of the devil and the attractiveness of the world are such that we Christians fall almost imperceptibly into confusing the treadmill with the ladder. We leave God out of our practical living. We do not consciously discipline ourselves to bring the Lord into everything we do.

Brother Lawrence, preparing the vegetables in the kitchen of a monastery in Paris in the seventeenth century, so 'practised the presence' of God that God was just as real to him among the vegetables and cooking pots as when he went into the chapel for the daily offices of worship. He has a lot to teach us. He turned his treadmill of domestic drudgery into a ladder leading to the presence of God.

Assuming God's interest to be limited

'*Whatever* you do, do *it all* for the glory of God' (1 Cor 10:31). So writes the apostle Paul to the Christians at Corinth – and he is talking about eating and drinking!

How seriously do we take his command? Put into practice it is the secret of a serene, steady ascent of the ladder of discipleship which God provides to raise us out of the cage. For the prevailing ethos in society – and in the church – is one in which the secular is separated from the sacred, and God is seen as being interested in one and not the other. The Lord may be involved in our Sunday and weekday worship and in our 'quiet times'; but in fact our *whole* life belongs to him. He is no less interested in our work, our leisure and our family life than he is in our services of worship, our prayer meetings, our Bible studies and our work around the church.

By making this unbiblical separation either consciously or unconsciously, and behaving accordingly, we confirm the world in its notion that God is quite irrelevant to ordinary human life. It is hardly surprising that most people think God an optional extra, an alternative way of spending leisure time. He is seen as an alternative to the weekend cottage, hang-gliding, the garden, DIY or the Sunday papers.

People can hardly be blamed for thinking that way when

so many Christians live as though God *was* simply a time-consuming leisure activity, rather than the Lord of all life, to whom the Christian is a bondslave sixty minutes an hour, twenty-four hours a day, seven days a week, fifty-two weeks a year, until his Lord calls him home. As George Herbert put it:

> Seven whole days, not one in seven,
> I will praise Thee;
> In my heart, though not in heaven,
> I can raise Thee.

This is a discipline of life, and has to be learnt and exercised. When we begin this way of total discipleship, then we shall begin to achieve spiritual and psychological integration; we shall be on the ladder not the treadmill, and the world will know because it will see the difference in us.

Deliberate displacement of God

When God has been excluded from one part of life, the slide into his becoming completely irrelevant is easy. Even if we continue to maintain habits of Christian behaviour, the life will seep from them and they will become what we have made them – mere habitual activities.

Once that has happened it is only a short step to the effective exclusion of God from any real role in our lives at all; we *live* as if God did not exist – what seventeenth-century pastors used to call 'practical atheism'. Open rejection of his claims can then so easily follow.

That is the way in which worldliness takes hold of the individual Christian in western society today, and also the pattern of the decline of Christianity in Europe. It is also why so many North American 'born-again Christians' are so vulnerable to the seductive ethos of the society in which they live.

The popularity and arrogance of unbelief

Modern man, confined within the cage, is proud of his understanding and achievements. He fails to see how limited his view really is, and the questions which have occupied the greatest minds of the past – those of meaning, purpose, the basis of morality, the transcendent, and beauty, truth and absolute values – are generally considered irrelevant, meaningless, or unanswerable.

Modern man is blinded to these aspects of life by his technological achievements, and deafened by the proclamation of the extent of his knowledge. He claims to be humble and objective in the face of the wonders of the universe. Nevertheless, by dismissing any source of knowledge outside of his own, finite, observations, he assumes a power of all-knowing which cannot possibly be his. Too often Christians easily slip into becoming children of their time.

G K Chesterton once observed that the church was the one thing that saved a man from the degrading servitude of being a child of his own time. Unfortunately, it is easy for Christians to bow to such degrading servitude, for associated with the arrogance of modern materialism of all kinds are values and attitudes which press us into the mould of this world. They can make short work of youthful devotion and zeal. How many zealous Christian students, on entering a career and the responsibilities of marriage, settle first for respectable support of a local church, then for attendance alone, because the pressures of life are so severe?

Respectable conformity has anaesthetized quite as many Christians as blatant immorality has strangled. They end up on the treadmill of selfish worldly activity, which ultimately leads nowhere, with only an occasional half-hearted jump in the general direction of the ladder. In the cage which shuts God out, they become as blind as the world to the reality outside, to which the ladder leads.

6
The results of worldly blindness

Men and women today live as though the only reality worth taking seriously is the cage in which, whether they realize it or not, they are imprisoned. Everything is decided in that context.

The ladder, even when it is pointed out to them, seems to lead only slowly to where they want to go; the treadmill is so much more inviting because it appears to lead much more readily to the summit of achievement. There seems to be no certainty that the ladder leads to where the rats on it say it does. How can we know that there *is* anything other than the cage? All we can see is the wire mesh marking the limits of that which we can appreciate with our senses. Beyond that all is dark and uncertain.

Modern man pretends that nothing exists beyond the limits of the cage, or that no one can really know anything about it, or that it doesn't really matter which way you move towards the cage's boundaries because in the end you will escape anyway.

The prostitution of work

Once the cage of the visible, material and finite world becomes the only reality, either by definite decision or simply by ignoring alternative views, then problems follow.

To begin with, work and activity become important for their own sake. That which should be done for the glory of God becomes an end in itself. My aims and their achievement then depend upon *my* efforts, *my* skills and *my* determination, rather than upon the grace and benevolence of God. Instead of my activity being totally consecrated to him, and therefore dependent upon him for its orientation and outcome, it becomes dependent on me.

Paul's exhortation, 'Whatever you do, do it all for the glory of God' (1 Cor 10:31) is one of the most practical and certainly the most health-giving words in scripture. It is at the core of the biblical ethic of work and life. Not to practise it is to prostitute the role that God intends work, both 'Christian' and 'secular', to play in our lives. It is just as easy to abuse God's gracious gift of work as it is to abuse his wonderful gift of sex.

The dehumanizing of man

Just as it applies to the individual, the prostitution of work characterizes human society, irrespective of political colour or ideological commitment. What should be a sacred dimension of human life becomes perverted and corrupted. Men become labour units. Those in management become expendable if they do not further the 'organization'. Those at the very top are in bondage to the desire for more money, power, influence or prestige, whether they recognize that as their deepest motive or not. Everyone is dehumanized. Different political systems and ideologies may have different structures, but the dehumanization is much the same. This is not to say that the individuals concerned are nasty people; many are very pleasant and altruistic, but they are none the less dehumanized, firmly chained to the treadmill, which in the end leads nowhere except to a more or less ornate box and six feet of earth – or consignment to the fire and a small urn of ashes. That is the end.

> This is the evil in everything that happens under the sun ['in the cage']: The same destiny overtakes all. The hearts of men, moreover, are full of evil and there is madness in their hearts while they live, and afterwards they join the dead. Anyone who is among the living has hope – even a live dog is better off than a dead lion! For the living know that they will die . . . this is your lot in life and in your toilsome labour under the sun ['in the cage'?] Whatever your hand finds to do, do it with all your might, for in the grave, where you are going, there is neither working nor planning nor knowledge nor wisdom . . . but the dead know nothing; they have no further reward, and even the memory of them is forgotten.' (Eccl 9:3–5a,9b,10,5b)

The oppression of the weak and poor

Inside the cage where ultimately all effort is futile, we are encouraged: 'Do everything with all your might in the hope that some satisfaction will be found in the transient achievement possible within such limits. There is no need to be too scrupulous about it, for the only way to get on is at the expense of others. If only a few can get to the top of the treadmill, they will have to do so on the backs of those lower down.' Thus we see everywhere in all cultures, in different ways, different contexts and to a greater or lesser degree, the oppression of the weak and the poor.

Even a revolution merely tips the top rats off the treadmill and installs some of the bottom ones at the top. There is still a hierarchy. The poor and weak are trodden under foot for the best of motives: in order to build a strong economy; or in order to pave the way for the Utopia which is only just around the next corner; or in order to defend our 'way of life', or our 'values', or our 'freedom', or our 'democratic system'; and so on. As Paul puts it: 'since they did not think it worth while to retain the knowledge of God, God has left them to their own irrational ideas' (Rom 1:28, NIV and conflated JB). No wonder the world is in a mess.

The arrogant use of power and wealth

Caught on the treadmill and unable to get off, the moral decline continues. The mill revolves more and more rapidly as those at the bottom increase their effort to get to the top, and those higher up work harder and harder to stay there. They increasingly discard principles and values, arrogantly using the power they find at the top to keep those lower down in their place. So, instead of a recognition of individual responsibility to God and to other human beings, a situation of inter-human conflict is created, in which the cry is all for 'human rights', individual and group; selected rights which are incompatable with others at many points.

The concept of 'human rights' is a valuable one but, without the complementary concept of responsibility to an outside authority, inter-group conflict is inevitable. Pressure groups with conflicting aims multiply. Such groups emerge and develop most often from the highest of motives, from sincere concern and true altruism. How sad that the good should turn so sour!

The devaluing of man; the overvaluing of things

Status on the treadmill, achieved at the cost of the dehumanization of oneself and others, is measured largely in terms of possessions and one's standard of living. Personal qualities of integrity, compassion, self-sacrifice and costly

service are no longer valued very much in themselves;
perhaps they never have been in society at large. The one
thing that counts is success. Things become more important
than people. As more people in society accumulate to themselves more wealth, what were once the sins of a small
number of the rich and prosperous become the sins of the
much larger group of the presently affluent.

Is this, in fact, where many of us find ourselves? Our
hearts are set on reaching the top of the mill, with little
real regard for our fellow rats or even concern about our
own rattiness! Our Lord warns us of the danger: 'Do not
store up *for yourselves* treasures on earth . . . where thieves
break in and steal. But store up for yourselves treasures in
heaven . . . For where your treasure is, there your heart
will be also' (Matt 6: 19–21). Interestingly, the security
industry is one of the growing points in all western econ-
omies. 'Do not be afraid', Jesus said,

> '..for your Father has been pleased to give you the
> kingdom. Sell your possessions and give to the poor.
> Provide purses for yourselves that will not wear out, a
> treasure in heaven that will not be exhausted, where no
> thief comes near and no moth destroys. For where your
> treasure is, there your heart will be also.'
>
> (Luke 12: 32–34)

The treasure which we are to lay up in heaven is that
righteousness which is the product of the work of the Holy
Spirit in our lives. His work is shown by love, joy, peace,
patience, kindness, goodness, trustfulness, gentleness and
self-control. How can these things be cultivated if our eyes
are firmly set on the top of the treadmill? Paul says: 'You
cannot belong to Christ Jesus unless you *crucify all self-
indulgent passions and desires*' (Gal 5:24, JB). God must grieve
at the ease with which his children conform – or are seduced
into conforming – to the ways of the world, when his
warnings are so very clear.

7
The symptoms of worldly blindness

The breakdown of ethics

We do not need to look very far to see the symptoms of a world-view that keeps God out of life. The breakdown of ethics in western society is one obvious example.

Perhaps Christians have majored too enthusiastically in recent years on the breakdown of sexual morality and the modification of the law in order to accommodate changing mores, to the exclusion of less obvious but no less significant features.

The breakdown of basic *integrity* is, to my mind, more alarming. To what extent can we rely on the word of another about anything significant, particularly concerning money or valuables? How many business deals and personal arrangements sidestep moral questions? How many decisions by governments, both national and local, are taken on purely fiscal grounds or on ideological premisses, rather than concern for the consequences in the lives of real people and real families? Yet basic integrity must be at the centre of all personal relationships and dealings if society is to be at all stable. Perhaps it has never been allowed this position, but Christians should be demonstrating it, even if it costs.

Our present tendency is to find ways of getting along comfortably in secular society (though we still recoil in horror at sexual sin). We give ourselves away by rationalizing and justifying our dubious plans, actions, and quite selfish ambitions and objectives.

Both my grandfathers had Christian integrity, and both were therefore prepared to take a costly stand on principle in their secular occupations.

One refused to put into practice certain instructions which he considered to be morally wrong, saying, 'To do that would be disloyalty to my Lord. What he requires is more important than keeping my job.' In the business he subsequently built he considered it his *Christian* responsibility to employ some who had been disabled in the 1914–18 war, not because legislation had been passed to force him to do so.

The other grandfather had been orphaned when he was nine and had educated himself while apprenticed as a joiner. He was deeply committed to the cause of social justice, and his life was devoted to the Labour movement in his local area. Yet he resigned from the management committee of his local co-operative society which he had helped to found, because of a dubious financial deal which they wished to cover up rather than expose. His comment in resigning was, 'If this movement is not built on absolute integrity, then its foundation is rotten, and it cannot stand. I can have no further part in it.'

I ask simply how many of us in positions of responsibility in business or the public service would be prepared to lose our jobs in order to maintain our Christian integrity? How many of us who are socially concerned or politically committed would resign, even though we knew that the exposure of a fundamental lack of honesty would damage a movement to which we were deeply and sincerely committed? If we do not have the same concern for absolute integrity and honesty in the situations in which we find ourselves today, then why not? Are we tied to the treadmill?

The breakdown of personal relationships

Without fundamental honesty and integrity, successful personal relationships cannot be built. Most of us have many acquaintances but few, if any, real friends. Our social relationships exist only at a superficial level. Far too often such real friendships as we do know are restricted to our own age group or class or profession. Even in the church where it should clearly not be so, friendship and sharing in integrity is largely horizontal (within the age groups) rather than vertical (through the age range). The excuse so often offered, *'They* don't really understand,' is an implicit confession of a lack of trust and a lack of love, which can be traced back to a fundamental lack of integrity between the individuals concerned. We grieve the Holy Spirit.

What is more, without deep personal relationships in real friendship we deny ourselves a major antidote to the stresses which lead to breaking-point, and also exclude a significant therapy if we do break under the strain. Friendship of that quality depends absolutely for its foundation upon real integrity, trust and responsibility. It is not common in society at large. The tragedy is that too often it is not present in the church either; the infection of worldliness has taken hold there too.

The search for satisfaction wholly within this life

Living within the cage means that if satisfaction at the personal level is to be achieved, it has to be within the confines of this present life, and without reference to God. Death is the great unspoken evil. The frustration of selfish fulfilment in this life is the supreme failure.

So on the one hand we see the frantic search for ways of prolonging life and, on the other, the advocacy of the right to terminate it by a deliberate act when it is no longer 'worth living'. Surely that is the grand irony, the supreme contradiction. In the world-view of modern western society we have created yet another tension for ourselves: we look for eternal fulfilment, but deny ourselves eternity.

The search for temporary escape

Many people are seeking refuge in the anaesthetics which are at present on offer: smoking, despite the known risks; alcohol, as a pick-me-up when there is a reason and increasingly when there is not; drugs, to open the door to another world. All these provide relief from the despair of real or imagined failure or uselessness, and from the inevitable pressures that success brings.

Vast sums of money are spent on the entertainment industry. The cost of maintaining television channels, the considerable investment in providing spectator sport, the world of pop, and no less the world of 'serious' music, visual art, theatre and cinema, are all part of the pattern of escape.

None of these things is bad in itself; they are all in a real sense good gifts of God to men, part of the distribution of his common grace. But perhaps the enormous sums involved should cause us to stop and ask whether they in fact form one extensive dispensary of pain-killers to help us cope with the pain of travelling fast and getting nowhere. Relaxation and enjoyment are good, and a necessary part of the life God intends men to lead, but when they become the most important dimension of life hasn't *something* gone wrong? Tranquillity, even the tranquillizer, is good and helpful in its place, but when tranquillizers become an addiction instead of a medication then we need to ask important questions.

Christians protest vigorously about the abuse of human sexuality which burgeons in our society. Promiscuity, adultery, fornication, soft and hard pornography, live sex shows, sexual abuse of children and young people, bestiality and all the rest have rightly been condemned. Certainly the heart of man is evil, but the growth of the sex industry is the result of a view of life which sees the cage as all there is. If this life is all we have to live for, the extension of our sensual experience is of paramount importance if we are to get the most out of life.

The search for self-realization

Much of the active preoccupation with sex in our society is possible only because of the increasing affluence in which we live out our lives, just as it was for some in the world of ancient Israel eight centuries before the coming of Christ. The sexual symptoms of moral laxity are rooted very deeply in the money-orientated life of the contemporary treadmill. They result from the breakdown of relationships mentioned earlier, and from the search for individual fulfilment.

This poses a real question for Christians. To what extent is the protest against permissiveness, right and proper in itself, an unconscious attempt to deflect attention from the real problems of worldliness in the *church*?

I suggest that we have two problems here. First, there is a subtle acceptance of the standards of the world in terms of domestic comfort and financial security. Our interest in both increases as we get older, and they become the norm within which and *for* which we work. And, second, large sections of evangelical Christianity in Europe and North America have been infected by the modern western ideal of individualism. Individual fulfilment has become the be-all and end-all of Christian experience. Salvation is, for us, simply a significant element in our search for self-fulfilment. We deny its right to embrace everything we have and all we are in the vital context of the people of God, outside whom there is no full salvation. Is it any wonder that so much corporate Christianity lacks real muscle and suffers from severe anaemia? Or that individuals within the group are subject to subtle tensions and ill-defined unease and pressure? Many are being torn between the ladder and the treadmill.

We, as Christians in the west, need to ask ourselves plainly and to answer honestly before God, some questions. Questions about ourselves and our attitude to life; about churches, especially our local congregation; about our lifestyle, priorities and ambitions; and about the kind of God we *really* worship and serve, and how he relates to our lives in *practice*, rather than theory.

How much of the doctrine we profess is merely a collection of shibboleths to sort out the 'sound' from the 'unsound' Christian? How much is really worked out in hard practical experience in the cage, but on the ladder rather than the mill? Intellectual belief alone achieves nothing. True faith *works*, and works in the hard grind of bitter and stressful experience in the cage. It transforms the life within it through the perspective it provides, and the hope which it offers.

PART THREE

In the race but not the cage:

God's people in the world

8
Sharing God's view

Realizing the reality of God

There are many obvious pressures on Christians in society, at work, and in their homes and churches. Such pressures are mostly inescapable in the world in which we find ourselves. The fact that some of us break under the strain, and many more lead grey and fraught Christian lives, is hardly surprising.

If however, we step outside the cage, even for a moment or two, and try to see the whole circus of frantic and largely fruitless activity as it really is, the bitter irony of it all is so very clear. Next to the apparently dynamic and, for some, successful activity on the treadmill, is a ladder with regular resting platforms which reaches higher than the mill and, at its end, leads to a world of freedom and light beyond the cage. But it is easier to pretend that there is nothing outside the cage, or that what lies outside is so uncertain that it can contribute nothing to our understanding of life within the cage. It is in the light of the transcendent reality of God, however, that the fundamental differences between the metaphorical ladder and the treadmill are shown up.

Relying on God's word in practice

If we are to escape from the treadmill and take up permanent residence on the ladder we need to learn to share God's perspective. That has to be done in practice as well as in theory. So many of us can know the theory backwards but when it comes to demonstrating real trust in the way we live and in our approach to life, our ceaseless round of busy and fraught activity shows how anxious we really are.

Yet our Lord said:

'Do not worry about your life, what you will eat or drink; or about your body, what you will wear . . . Who of you by worrying can add a single hour to his life? . . . So do not worry . . . For the pagans run after all these things, and your heavenly Father knows that you need them. But seek first his kingdom and his righteousness, and all these things will be given to you as well. Therefore do not worry about tomorrow . . .'

(Matt 6:25,27,31–34)

The apostle Peter also wrote:

'Cast all your anxiety on him because he cares for you.'
(1 Pet 5:7)

This is not just good advice to be taken and put into practice; it is a *command* to be obeyed – from our Lord as well as his apostle.

Recently we received a letter from a missionary friend in

Africa. She is chronically ill, and the control of her disease depends upon the availability of a regular supply of the appropriate drugs. She is in a lonely outpost running a dispensary in an area that often suffers from drought. Basic necessities are often in short supply and she had been burgled while away for a rest in a more congenial part of the country. The first sentence of the letter was one of praise to God. And the second quoted the verse from Peter, and commented, 'I have learnt that anxiety is a sin.' Of course it is, because it is disobedience. But how many of us treat it in that way? Even if we admit it, how seriously do we treat it? Do we put it on the same level as if we had committed fornication or adultery – or murder? What is the answer? Greater resolution and effort in fighting anxiety? Resisting every fear and worry? Not primarily, though effort may be required. Before Peter makes the statement already quoted, he writes:

' "God opposes the proud but gives grace to the humble" [quoting from Prov 11:31]. Humble yourselves, therefore, under God's mighty hand, that he may lift you up in due time.'

(1 Pet 5:5–6)

The first and greatest requirement is for us to recover our vision of God's greatness, and to live by it. Many, perhaps most, of us are simply too proud and self-sufficient to humble ourselves under the mighty hand of God. We want God to be the great problem-solver when things get beyond us. We want to bring God in on the big decisions, at least in theory. We want him to take over at the point when we can no longer cope from our own resources.

In God's eyes that is not good enough. He wants us to live every dimension of our lives at every level *under his mighty hand*, from the most important and fundamental aspects to the most insignificant detail. That, ultimately, is what using the ladder of discipleship means.

One Christmas, a Nigerian friend stayed with us. He told

us of the problems of obtaining even the necessities of life, and of the unreliability of basic services like a water supply and electricity, kerosene, and petrol and tyres for the car. He added, 'but it is good, because you have to pray to the Lord for everything!'

How many of us 'pray to the Lord for everything'? That is part of what it means to humble ourselves under God's mighty hand. It is only by doing so that we do, in fact, 'cast our anxiety' on him – but it is no good waiting until we are on the verge of a breakdown before we start to practise that.

It is significant that the apostle Peter addresses these commands specifically to *young* men. The practice of the presence of God is a discipline that ought to begin in youth. That is the greatest safeguard against breakdown later in life.

Most of us find it easy to accept that God is great and glorious. We look to the glory of the sky on a starry night and say with the psalmist:

'When I consider your heavens, the work of your fingers . . . what is man that you are mindful of him, the son of man that you care for him?'

(Ps 8:3,4)

But we fail to go on with the psalmist to wonder at the position God has given man in relation to the rest of his creation. We fail to take seriously enough the fact that God *is* interested in us and *does* care for us.

Someone said to me recently, 'I feel so very embarrassed when I try to bring the Lord into my very minor problems; surely it's too much to expect him to be concerned with them, when there are so many other Christians with much greater problems than I have?' Why 'embarrassed'? God is even interested when his children go bald! Didn't Jesus say that the individual hairs on our heads are all *counted*? Luke sets the saying in the context of God's *care:*

'Are not five sparrows sold for two pennies? Yet not one of them is forgotten by God. Indeed, the very hairs of your head are all numbered. Don't be afraid; you are worth more than many sparrows.'

(Luke 12:6,7)

God is great in that his knowledge and care embrace not only the unimaginable vastness of space, but also each individual elementary particle which atomic physicists have yet to discover in the nucleus of the atom. It is *that* God who cares for us, his children. We have no need to doubt his power, knowledge or love. There is every reason to take *every* aspect of our lives to him, and make that total commitment a habit.

To practise the presence of God is to live every part of our lives willingly and consciously in his presence. To be on the ladder is to be fully incorporated into the total purpose of God. It is only in this way that we can be at peace with God, not only in the sense of being fundamentally right with him in the sense of 'justification', but also in our daily walk with him.

Step-by-step obedience to God is the expression of our love for him. So often we think of that obedience only in terms of major decisions and acts, but it refers to *all* we do. My love for my wife is expressed not only in the fact that we work together in major things, but that over thirty-two years of marriage we have increasingly learnt to work together in small things as well – in all the quite ordinary activities which are of the essence of life. It is the same with our relationship to God in Christ by his Spirit.

When did you last commit a boring detail of your work to God, consciously and deliberately? Or the routine events of life, like travelling to work, doing the shopping? What about those household chores, some of which at least even working husbands ought to share? When did you last commit the pleasures of life to God – being with the family, going out with the children, listening to music, relaxing in front of your favourite television programme?

A right view of the importance of this life

It is all too easy to become so preoccupied with this life and its concerns that we fail to see it in the light of God's purposes. We become too earthly-minded to seek any heavenly good. But, on the other hand, it is just as easy to be so preoccupied with 'spiritual' things that we fail to see the importance of the life we are called to lead on this earth. We become too heavenly-minded to be any earthly good.

The safeguard against both mistakes is not to try to achieve some kind of balance between them, but to bring the Lord into everything that we do. That way the *whole* of life comes under his control, from the greatest decision and the most intractable problem to the most insignificant act and the smallest irritation.

The need to persevere

The greatest saints of God have practised his presence and learnt the secret of godliness with contentment. Apart from such complete and confident submission in every part of his life, Paul could not have written:

'I have *learned* to be content whatever the circumstances. I know what it is to be in need, and I know what it is to have plenty. I have *learned* the secret of being content in any and every situation, whether well fed or hungry, whether living in plenty or in want. I can do everything through him who gives me strength.'

(Phil 4:11–13, italics mine)

'*Learning*' implies progression and perseverance, discipline and determination. The contentment did not come as a sudden transformation, or by a miraculous visitation of the Spirit. It was a process of learning by experience, as the apostle makes clear in Romans 5:1–5. Are we prepared to learn and to discipline ourselves? It is the only way to that contentment which acts as a sea wall against the pressures that can bring us to breaking-point. It is not, however, an easy road; it takes determination and perseverance. Paul's words were written at the end of his life, but I wish that I had seen my life in that perspective when I was younger so that later on the accumulating pressures would have been recognized and dealt with more easily.

Living in the context of God's eternal purpose

To realize the greatness of God and the goodness and certainty of his purpose is also to bring another perspective to bear on stress and pressure. For, if I walk with him, I am working out my life in the context and framework of his purpose. My responsibility is to obey; his promise is to work all things together for my good and for the good of all his people (Rom 8:28–30).

Never divorce that promise from its context, which is the gracious and good purpose of the omnipotent God, whose love has been set upon you quite deliberately. Never restrict the promise. The '*all* things' in which 'God works for the good of those who love him' *means all things*. Even the sins and shortcomings, the deviations from his way and the disobedience to his will. The Christian who looks back on his life will regret the many times he strayed from the way, but he will see that God used even the longest and most distant detours to *his* glory and therefore the blessing of his disciple.

The actual pathway taken step by step is less important than the direction in which we move. The pathway is only the way by which we attain the goal upon which we must keep our eyes fixed. As we continue to climb the ladder of discipleship towards the ultimate goal of being 'conformed to the image of Christ' our stumbling and hesitant steps will become increasingly certain, steady and determined as the goal becomes more clear. When we slip a rung we shouldn't set about a morbid dissection of how terribly guilty we are. Our guilt has already been dealt with by Christ and 'the blood of Jesus goes on purifying us from every sin' (1 John 1:7, literal rendering).

If we *walk in the light*, that is, opening ourselves completely to the scrutiny of the Holy Spirit, our attitude to sins committed after we become God's children should be simple: admit them before God, and forget them. The proper reaction to sin and failure, and the way to use them in Christian growth, is to *learn* from them so that we do not fall into the same trap again. Of course, the Lord's enemy and our own desires will produce plenty more different traps, but as we begin to recognize traps – or slippery rungs – we shall begin to get the measure of our enemy. That will be true growth; real progress up the ladder.

We need to remember, though, that we are on a ladder, and not strapped into a rocket. There is no easy route to the goal of being like Jesus. Yet for all of us there will be times when we feel that God has gently lifted us up a few rungs. That serves to assure us that he really cares and is involved in our stumbling progress. It is not to make us think there is an easier way – if not a rocket then a hot air balloon – to save us the effort of moving more or less steadily upwards rung by rung. Reliance on hot air is not to be recommended; the burner fails sooner or later. Unfortunately there is a lot of hot air around in the church today. In confusing this with the real and gracious lift of the invisible hand of God, God's people are deluded into thinking that they have reached the top of the ladder.

Our susceptibility to stress and breakdown will be greatly affected by the way we live our lives in the normal course of events, not only when we reach the age at which we might expect to come under special pressure. The younger we are when we begin to live our lives God's way, and discipline ourselves into godly habits of thought and action, the more we shall be garrisoned against future pressure and stress. Certainly we all have different genetic make-ups and different histories, but these, too, are under God's all-powerful grace and purpose. He understands and knows each of us and he helps each of us as our personal needs dictate.

We need to recover our vision of the greatness and love of God, and live as though it were real! We need to see our lives, down to the smallest detail, as having a part in his eternal, universal, cosmic purpose, and live in the light of the certainty of his interest and care for everything that concerns us. We need to practise his presence and to persevere in his path for us; to rely on what he is and upon what he has said in his word, however we feel. We need to trust when his presence is not felt, and rejoice when we are specially conscious of it.

Our activity – the obverse of the Holy Spirit's working in our lives

We must learn to bring God into every part of our lives. All that we do should be the obverse of the activity of God's Spirit. Our life is not a self-contained, unaided, personal effort on our part – a closed system into which we choose to let God at certain points and at certain times. It is a continuing response of active faith (and there isn't any other kind of faith!) to what God is, to what he has promised, and to what he has in fact done for us in the Lord Jesus Christ.

In active faith the sacred and the secular cannot be separated without the risk of developing spiritual schizophrenia – which is a major cause of stress, pressure and breakdown. Such a separation, conscious or unconscious, is in fact a continual jumping from the treadmill to the ladder and back again.

Let's face facts. All that we have – salary, wages, home, possessions, security, career, prospects – ultimately come from God, and he gives or withholds as he sees best for our ultimate good. We are to use his gifts in personal responsibility to him. They are not ours by right; we do not deserve them. If we have worked hard for them, the strength and health to do so have been given by God. So we should be able to relax, leaving the outcome of our work in his good hands, and walking in daily obedience and trust. If he takes away some, or all, of these gifts, even then we can trust him and seek his blessing.

Openness for sacrifice

The first thing we need to do in order to leave the treadmill and start back on the ladder is to sacrifice to God on the altar all that we have been given, all that we have achieved, all that we enjoy, all that we rely on, and all that we hope for – perhaps also all that we fear, now or for the future. In God's hands it is in safe keeping and can be enjoyed and used by us without fretting or idolatry or concern.

For most keen, active Christians, often the first thing that needs to be laid on the altar of sacrifice is their Christian service. It is valuable service only if it is done genuinely in service of God, rather than in service of one's career or ego. There is far too much 'carnal' or self-centred service of God in his church and the organizations associated with it. If you doubt that just try to change the patterns of activity in the local church! The protective fence goes up immediately. That is the surest sign of carnal service on the part of the fencing contractors.

The test of spiritual service is that, like Isaac, born by the promise of God and a miracle of his grace, it is laid out on the altar. The knife is raised ready to be plunged deep into its heart, in the belief that God is able and ready to raise up a new work, to his greater glory, out of the death of the old. The test that shows if the work we do for God is in fact the work of God, is *not* that we are prepared to cut it out if God leads us so to do, rather that we will stop the work *unless God commands us to continue*.

Try the test with your contribution to the work of the church – your Bible class, your Crusader, Covenanter or Campaigner group, your youth club, your choir or music group, your position as organist or director of music, your preaching and teaching, and your leading of worship. Unless the lethal knife is often and regularly raised over our activities they will become more self-centred and less God-centred. The more this happens the more stress and pressure we bring on ourselves, because we are trying to do *God's* work in our *own* strength.

The way to counter this is to make worship central and all-pervading. We need to learn in a new way, or learn again, the practical secret that it is in the process of being worshipped that God communicates his presence to us. God's presence is absolutely essential if 'Christian' activity is to be *God's* work. Work and activity in which God is not present, however well organized, Bible-based, numerically successful or admirable, is not God's work.

Those of us in active evangelical churches often moan about the lack of results from our well-prepared and wide-ranging activities. Why do these young people either disappear from our congregations when they reach their late teens, or settle down into mere churchgoing when they get married? Maybe the sacrificial knife needs some ruthless wielding by our church and youth leaders. That will be done only as we concentrate more and more on God in worship, allowing the painful presence of God to be felt in our individual and corporate lives and to prune out the useless aspects of our work for him. We would see a deep transformation of our lives and church communities which would be a real work of God.

The problem is that many Christians who have success-fully got off one treadmill merely transfer to another – that of 'Christian activity'. May God give us the grace to distinguish between this and the ladder of true discipleship.

9
Sharing with the people of God

The need for true worship

As we have seen, there is a great need for us to experience true worship and to see its real importance. The wartime Archbishop of Canterbury, William Temple, wrote: 'This world can be saved from political chaos and collapse by one thing only, and that is worship.'

It is not only the world that needs saving, the church does too. The chaos produced by so many self-perpetuating interest groups within the local congregation will not be resolved simply by removing them all. The devising of a more efficient system of organization and intercommunication won't help either.

The answer will only be found in a concentration on worship. The strained structures do not need better bolts, new techniques of construction or more highly trained technicians, but a rediscovery of the true foundation of the building.

What is worship? William Temple defined it beautifully:

'To worship is
to quicken the conscience by the holiness of God,
to feed the mind with the truth of God,
to purge the imagination by the beauty of God,
to open the heart to the love of God,
to devote the will to the purpose of God.'

Worship is a total orientation towards God which offers to him all that we have and are. In worship God transforms us for his use. That is the secret of true and effective service. We do not offer him our plans, our ideas, our programmes, our organizations, and ask him to bless them; we offer him *ourselves*. Having done that, the programmes and the organizations are then his full responsibility as we work them out in active cooperation with him. This applies at both the individual and corporate levels.

Worship – a priority commitment

What does the recovery of worship involve?

Primarily it implies that worship will encompass *all* levels of our lives, not only our individual devotions, which most keen Christians recognize to be of real importance.

In the family

How many Christian families gather together for regular worship, not necessarily daily but at least once a week? Worship is putting God at the centre, not only in theory but also in practice. God must be *seen* to be at the centre. We see children brought up in Christian homes rejecting the faith and deserting the Christ to whom they have been introduced. How many do so because at root they detect hypocrisy in their family life? They see a Christianity which is preoccupied with activity and neglects worship. Christian families must learn to value and to practise corporate worship. Christians on the ladder of discipleship are not climbing as individuals; they progress together, and for many the main communal unit is the family.

In groups within the church

Consider also groups within the church itself. The house group has done a great deal to recover one dimension of corporate worship; but what of the other groups into which our congregations so readily divide? Choirs might well begin their regular practice with a reading from scripture and a time of prayer. Yet how many are content with a perfunctory prayer as a prelude to the 'real' business, or with nothing at all? The same question should be asked of all the many groups which meet regularly on our church premises – of youth organizations and clubs, of the committees and leaders' groups, of senior citizens' groups, women's guilds, and so on.

This failure is a symptom of the disease that afflicts the twentieth-century western church. We live in the age of the schizophrenic church: we have separated elements which should be united – worship from activities, sacred pursuits from secular ones, work from prayer, social action from preaching the gospel. Is it then any wonder that so many of those who take positions of leadership break under the strain? How many churches are tearing their clergy and other leaders apart?

Everything that the individual Christian and the local church engages in should be *worship* in the sense so eloquently set out by William Temple. It should be a response to the holiness, the truth, the beauty, the love, and the purpose of God, and should be *seen* to be so. *All* that we do should be inspired, initiated, planned, permeated, empowered by and wholly subject to, God himself, by the working of his Spirit. Anything that is not is futile. As churches and as individuals we need to let *that* light penetrate our world-dulled minds.

In the whole church

What, then, of the worship of the *whole* church, both that of the local congregation and that of the people of God worldwide? Has this any relevance to the lifting of pressure and stress? It is of supreme significance at a number of levels. For example, what part does the corporate prayer of the whole church play in the life of your local church? Is it restricted to a few rather shallow and uninformed intercessions at Sunday worship? Is it only the faithful few (who are often seen as those who have little better to do in terms of servicing organizations) who gather in a small room once a week to pray for the work of the church, their prayers often accompanied by the din of yet another activity taking place in the next room? This should be the most important meeting of the week at which all those active in the work of the church are present, both to lay their burden of responsibility before the whole church and to share in prayer for the work in which they and others are involved. Prayer is the living root of everything else – of the preaching of the word, the right use of the sacraments, and the response to both in the worship, prayer, work and witness of God's people. It is the power and dynamic of evangelism, of Christian social action, and of active concern for the world which God has created.

In the record of the early church there are many examples in which the meeting of the church for prayer is either recorded or clearly implied. The church waits for God's guidance (Acts 1:14); seeks God's direction for right decisions (1:24–25); waits for the coming of the Spirit of God in power (2:1); meets for corporate worship, which included prayer (2:42); asks for the power of the Holy Spirit (4:24–31); lays a special responsibility for prayer upon leaders and office-bearers (6:2–4); commissions for service (6:6); seeks the power of the Holy Spirit for new converts (8:15); approves family prayer and worship (10:2); receives God's guidance through prayer (10:9–20; cf 8:26–40); intercedes for a leader in danger (12:5); makes prayer a constant feature of its life (12:12); chooses and commissions for missionary work (13:2–3); chooses and commissions for oversight and administration (14:23); displays active concern for missionary service (15:40); uses the prayer meeting as the place of conversion (16:13–15); finds the prayer meeting a place of witness and a source of miracles (16:25–34); and the meeting is the place of mutual commitment at a time of parting (20:36–38).

In each of these instances the setting is either the corporate prayer of the whole church gathered together or of a significant group within it. There is scarcely a dimension of the life and activity of the church which is not covered by these instances.

We sing, 'Prayer is the Christian's vital breath, the Christian's native air . . .' It is also the vital breath and native air of Christ's body, the church. Group prayer, and pre-eminently the church prayer meeting, is the lung of the church. The word of God, read, learnt and inwardly digested, is her food; worship her exercise; and evangelism and service her work. None of these can be effective without the vital breath.

The need for wide Christian fellowship

The corporate prayer of the whole church is the great leveller. It is an activity in which *all* may participate, regardless of age, occupation, status in the church or outside it, or any other difference. Not all have to contribute by articulated prayer, though some must, for all can join in silently as the Spirit moves one and another to lead.

God, however, has his way of giving us words and the courage to speak them. I know a church where six- and seven-year-old children pray simply, in the presence of 100 to 150 people at the prayer meeting. That meeting lasts two and a half hours, though most family groups leave after an hour and a half or so. The children are *not* bored or distracting; they truly participate. It is in such meetings of the church that the reality of the outside of the cage, and the fact that the ladder leads to it, are most clearly recognized, indeed seen and experienced.

There are, of course, bad prayer meetings as well as good ones. Leading a meeting for prayer requires as much practical and spiritual preparation as leading worship or preaching. Good prayer meetings do not just happen, any more than inspiring worship just happens. Both require preparation, not only on the part of the leader, but also by those who come. Effective prayer needs *information*, which has to be collected, collated, and digested for succinct presentation to the meeting. It needs *imagination*, so that those who participate can put themselves into the situations about which they pray. It also requires *inspiration*, which can come only from the Holy Spirit. All three presuppose *preparation* on the part of all who come. Bad prayer meetings usually result from ineffective leadership or inadequate preparation, or from a combination of both.

That there seem to be so many poor prayer meetings is but another symptom of the fact that the church has lost her way in relation to the centrality of worship and the Godward dimension of her activity. Think, for example, of the time and effort that goes into planning and preparing youth activities. Then compare it with time and effort that goes into preparing for a meeting for corporate prayer. Is it any wonder that some find such meetings boring and embarrassing? They then feel guilty because they know they ought to meet for prayer, and pressure and stress from another direction begin to accumulate. We need to pray, with the disciples, 'Lord, teach us to pray'.

The need for wide Christian awareness

It is in such meetings for prayer that we can be challenged and encouraged by our recognition of the fact that we are a part of a company which no man can number: the church worldwide and the church glorified in God's presence as well as militant here on earth.

In corporate prayer individuals can keep the whole group informed in detail about the needs, achievements and hopes of the people of God elsewhere. This helps us to see our own work in a new perspective. Our failures and achievements, our problems and our encouragements, our material and our spiritual life, all begin to fall into place as we learn of, and consider and pray for, the people of God worldwide. Our tunnel vision is increasingly widened as we enter into their problems, encouragements, achievements and failures. We *know* that our prayers are effective. For the Spirit and the Son make intercession for us and aid us in our feebleness and inadequacy (Rom 8:26,27; Heb 9:24).

As you have read these past pages you may have felt that worship and prayer have been emphasized to excess, and that their relevance to stress and pressure is limited. In fact you may think we have digressed quite unforgivably from the subject of this book! But it is important to remember here that we are concerned with prevention, with the avoidance of breakdown under the stress and pressure of life in western society and in the church today. Diagnosis and analysis of the underlying causes are therefore inevitable.

Early in the book we noted that non-Christian psychiatrists are not far wrong when they point to the church and Christian involvement there as a cause of chronic depression in Christians. As I reflect on my own breakdown I have to admit that such an observation would have been, to a significant degree, quite justified. Further reflection has led me to see that the stress and pressure in my church life came from two sources. First, from wrong attitudes and misplaced protest; second, from the structures and activity patterns within which I was working in the local church. This is no criticism of the individuals with whom I was working; Christians are caught up in structures and patterns by historical accident and live and work in churches that have lost their sense of direction.

Our other problems – confusing philosophy with theology, developing social action as an end in itself, making doctrine largely an intellectual concept rather than a transforming power for the whole person – would begin to fall back into place if we were to recover our vision of God in worship.

This is the New Testament pattern, as it was clearly the pattern laid down for the people of God in the Old Testament. Their deliverance from Egypt by the saving grace of God was designed to produce in them a life of individual and corporate obedience centred on, and empowered by, their fellowship with him in worship. God provided a way by which his government, leadership and control would have become a practical reality. Because of the fact of his power and love, the work he gave them to do should have been accomplished effectively and without stress (though not without effort) because he would accomplish it through them. That is still his way.

The real God whom we seek has revealed himself as one who is at work today. He wants to be involved in even the smallest details of the lives of his children, and in the corporate life of his people in all their activity in this world, so that they may become part of his purpose in everything that they do. It is the personal and corporate discipline of working this out in daily living that safeguards against the pressures of life, both outside and inside the church. The sooner that begins for every Christian, the stronger the defence against pressure and stress becomes.

The way back

Individually, it is up to us. As congregations of God's people, the change is much more complicated. Maybe the route back to the right path has to be slow and sure. A church may need its forty years in the wilderness to teach it to rely wholly on the Lord. I sometimes wonder, though, what would happen if some time, somewhere, a local church saturated with all kinds of good Christian activities were to call a halt to them all, literally cancelling *everything except* corporate worship and corporate prayer. The clear-out would include the choir and any other special group, even if it made a contribution to worship. Then, having pared everything down to that bare minimum, God would be allowed to lead the whole congregation through the worship and prayer, and to reveal the gifts he has given to them. Through the same prayer and worship, the Lord would then lead into the use of those gifts according to his will. There would then need to be constant openness, through prayer and worship, to a continuing pattern of transformation and change.

I am well aware that there are Christian groups who say that this is precisely what they have done by breaking away from the established mainstream denominations. My knowledge of many such groups is that they show an even greater tendency to rapid ossification than have the mainstream groups. Free worship can be just as much a bondage to pattern as a fixed liturgy. Perhaps the freedom that tends towards anarchy is, in fact, the greatest bondage (see, for instance, 1 Cor 14:20–32.)

The main point is quite clear. Prevention is preferable to cure. The way we run our churches today is in itself a pressure, producing stress in those who are most devoted and active within those structures. Until we recover the vision of a church which is a worshipping, interconnected and interdependent body, then those pressures will remain and the ladder of discipleship will be subtly transformed into a treadmill of frantic activity within the church itself. A transformed church would produce an environment in which the individual could do more than simply be released from some of the pressures of life. It would facilitate personal and individual discipline and growth in the Christian life, and provide an additional defence against the pressures which come inevitably from outside the church.

A pilgrim people

The society in which we live is very largely pagan, in practice if not in profession, and from the top levels to the bottom. Some surveys show that seventy per cent of British people believe in God. But ask those same people what difference that professed belief makes to the way they actually live and, for most, the honest answer would have to be 'nothing'. Yet Christians are always 'aliens, strangers and pilgrims' in this world, seeking a permanent residence only in the city of God (Heb 11:8–10,13–16;13:13–14). We are God's pilgrim people in a plastic society.

When we begin to live as though we were pilgrims rather than permanent residents, we shall start to remove much of the strain which comes from trying to achieve permanence in this life alone. The verses in Hebrews which have been referred to show precisely what living like that means in practice. For us, it will require reappraisal of our church and individual life along the lines suggested. May God grant that we begin to get to grips with these issues.

Sadly the church in which we have to live and work is not at all what God would have it to be – and never has been, even in New Testament times. We have to live in the church and world as they are, while holding always to the vision of what they might be by God's grace. How do we do that? To that we must now turn.

PART FOUR

Turning the treadmill into a ladder:

advice for Christian rats

10
Under pressure in the Old Testament

Our problems are not new. The biblical record contains many examples of pressure and stress – and of those who have come to breaking-point under it. The scriptures are given for our instruction, so that we can learn from those examples which God has caused to be recorded. Here, of course, we shall have to be selective in whose lives we look at.

Elijah

Consider, for example, the prophet Elijah (1 Kings 19). God had used him in a spectacular way, had preserved him through drought and famine, and had given him supreme courage in speaking the word of God to Ahab and Jezebel.

His evangelistic success had apparently been quite
dramatic. The forces of evil had been routed, and there had
been a mass return to the worship of Yahweh. Yet at the
mere threat of Jezebel (2) he is reduced to the deepest
depression; 'I have had enough, Lord. Take my life; I am
no better than my ancestors' (4). Why did he feel that way?
We can see from the way God dealt with him.

First, God provided food and rest (5–7). Elijah was physically exhausted, and had neglected his basic bodily needs.
He had driven himself in God's service to the point of utter
physical extremity; and God met that need first.

That is lesson one for us. We have no need to drive
ourselves physically to the point of breakdown. We need
to provide for our bodily requirements, and we need to
learn to relax and rest physically. Sometimes, of course,
God does require superhuman efforts from us in his service,
but if he requires it then he provides special grace to
meet it. But that is not his normal demand. Too often our
driving of ourselves is our own decision because we,
perhaps quite subconsciously, think God's work depends
upon us, and that he cannot do without us. At one level
that is true, for we all have our unique part to play in his
purpose, but that purpose does not depend ultimately upon
our efforts.

God then removed Elijah from the scene of his activity.
Physically strengthened and relaxed, he is sent into the
wilderness for a long period (8) where he finds further rest
(9). He had to learn the value of a break from fraught and
frenzied activity; a period in which God could speak to
him.

Lesson number two is that we need to make time to meet
with God, and to hear him speak to us. This links back to
our consideration of the centrality of prayer and worship,
both individual and corporate, and self-discipline. We all
acknowledge the need for this, but how many of us practise
it? It is squeezed out by the activity with which we so easily
fill our waking hours. Yet without that discipline of time,

we bring ourselves closer to breaking-point. Ask yourself what proportion of your time is spent in prayer and worship before God, and how much in frantic effort *doing* things for God. If the laity discount the time spent in legitimate activities associated with work and home, what answer do they give? If clergy and full-time lay workers ask the same question about their whole allocation of time, what answer can they give?

In the wilderness God asked his prophet, in effect, 'What are you doing in this state?' (9). Elijah's reply is revealing: 'I have been very zealous for the Lord but all my efforts have come to nothing: that lot who were so recently enthusiastic have turned against your prophets. I am the only one left and they are after me too!' (10). He was preoccupied with his own efforts, with what *he* had done, with *his* enthusiasm, devotion and perseverance. It was all true, he had indeed been zealous for the Lord; but he was looking inwards and relying on his qualities and efforts for the results instead of being content to leave the outcome to God.

Lesson three is that we are in danger when we become preoccupied with *our* patch in the church, with the work *we* do for the Lord, instead of with *God himself*. We need constantly to pray, to paraphrase the words of John Paul II, 'Preserve me from becoming so occupied with the work of the Lord that I neglect the Lord of the work.' We need not only to pray, but to watch closely as well.

Then the Lord ordered him to go out on to the mountain. Here called Horeb, the mountain was formerly known as Sinai, the place where God had revealed himself to his people. But God did not choose to reveal himself this time through the spectacular signs of wind, earthquake and fire. His presence was revealed only by a gentle whisper in Elijah's ear (11, 12). Hearing that voice, Elijah hid his face (13) and went to the mouth of the cave, ready to hear God speak again. The Lord repeated his former question, and Elijah his grumble.

Lesson four is that we must not look for the presence of

God only in the spectacular, in signs and wonders, but also, perhaps generally, in the steady, silent, almost mundane signs of his activity, which only the truly discerning can perceive. God is there, whether we feel his presence or not; and his gentle whisper to us is as sure a demonstration of his presence as the most dramatic demonstration of his power and grace. If our trust in God depends on seeing signs – which, though part of God's working are by no means all of it – we shall again be heading for breaking-point as the pressure to seek them becomes more and more urgent.

What does God *say* to Elijah? He does not give him a direct solution. He says, 'Go back the way you came' (15), 'Go back to the place where I have put you to serve me, and continue to work there.' For Elijah there was no escape from the work which God had given him, no retirement or move to a new location away from the pressures which he felt so deeply.

There is our fifth lesson: we cannot escape pressures by opting out of the work God has given to us, or by moving to another church. We shall only move from one set of pressures to another. Those which we experience in the place where God has set us have to be faced as they are and, if we are where he wants us to be, his strength will be ours to meet them.

Sometimes it seems to me that loyalty is a virtue which is fast disappearing. Many seem to leave a church and move on to another for the most trivial of reasons – the hymn book that is used, the vicar's manner or voice, the use of modern music – or its not being used! – and so on. Perhaps the only valid reason for moving on is that it would be sin before God to stay. God's answer to Elijah was not to transfer him to another cage, but to put him back on the same ladder on which he had been before he jumped on to the treadmill the devil so temptingly placed next to the ladder.

It is almost as an afterthought that God points to the fact that Elijah was wrong anyway – there were in fact 7,000 who were faithful to the Lord, besides Elijah. He was not on the ladder alone (18). To emphasize this, God gave him a companion and successor to continue the work – the first thing Elijah had to do was to anoint Elisha. How gracious God is!

There, too, is a lesson for us. Not only do we do his work in company with others, but God has already chosen and appointed those who will continue his work into the future when we have passed on to our reward; and they are already with us to be nurtured and trained in the ways of God. It is the prayer of an old rat who has made many mistakes by jumping from the ladder to the treadmill – and who eventually fell off – that his experience will be useful to the younger rats who will continue the work.

Jeremiah

So much for Elijah. What of Jeremiah? A very different character – diffident and shy, rather introverted and sensitive. Not only that, he was also a very young man when God called him to what was perhaps the most thankless task God can call anyone to: to preach God's word to a people who will not only choose to ignore it, but actually fight against the word and the messenger. God told Jeremiah that would happen before he had spoken a word to the people.

Jeremiah had been brought up in the closeted atmosphere of a priestly family in Judah. He had a deep sense of his own inadequacy, but God gave him a message of judgment for the people of Judah. His word from God was not one that offered to hold back his chastising anger in response to repentance; rather he was to tell them that the way to salvation was to be *through* judgment. Because that judgment was to take the form of conquest and slavery by Nebuchadnezzar's hordes from the east, Jeremiah's message of acceptance had severe political implications. His message seemed to Judah and its leaders to be the mouthings of a traitor, and they treated him as such.

It is hardly surprising that Jeremiah found his ministry to a faithless people an agony. Despite the promise of ultimate restoration he cried in desperation to God:

> 'Since my people are crushed, I am crushed;
>   I mourn, and horror grips me . . .
> Oh, that my head were a spring of water
>   and my eyes a fountain of tears!
> I would weep day and night
>   for the slain of my people.'
>
> (Jer 8:21–9:1)

But he was submissive to the will of God, however hard and bitter to his soul it might be:

> 'I know, O Lord, that a man's life is not his own;
>   it is not for man to direct his steps.'
>
> (Jer 10:23)

He could not understand why God allows the wicked to prosper, when he is prepared to punish his own people for their sin:

> 'You are always righteous, O Lord,
>   when I bring a case before you.
> Yet I would speak with you about your justice:
>   Why does the way of the wicked prosper?'
>
> (Jer 12:1)

The Lord does not answer Jeremiah's question, but tells him to trust that God knows what he is doing. Further, God forbids Jeremiah even to pray for the people of God:

> 'Do not pray for the well-being of this people. Although they fast, I will not listen to their cry; though they offer burnt offerings and grain offerings, I will not accept them. Instead, I will destroy them . . .'
>
> (Jer 14:11, 12; see also 7:16; 11:14.)

This drives the perplexed prophet to ask more questions

about God's purposes (14:13). The reply is that God is punishing persistent rebellion (16:10–13), but that he will restore the repentant (16:14,15;17:7, 8). Jeremiah then worships the God he knows, serves and loves:

> 'A glorious throne, exalted from the beginning,
>   is the place of our sanctuary.
> O Lord, the hope of Israel,
>   all who forsake you will be put to shame . . .
>   they have forsaken the Lord,
>   the spring of living water.
> Heal me, O Lord, and I shall be healed;
>   save me and I shall be saved,
>   *for you are the one I praise.*'

(Jer 17:12–14)

He pleads, as proof of his own repentance, his faithfulness to his commission (17:16). There is only the barest trace of self-pity as he considers the catch–22 situation in which he finds himself:

> ' . . . the word of the Lord has brought me
>   insult and reproach all day long.
> But if I say, "I will not mention him
>   or speak any more in his name,"
> his word is in my heart like a fire,
>   a fire shut up in my bones.
> I am weary of holding it in;
>   indeed, I cannot.'

(Jer 20:8, 9)

His confidence in God reasserts itself:

> 'But the Lord is with me like a mighty warrior . . .
> Sing to the Lord!
>   Give praise to the Lord!'

(Jer 20:11, 13)

But almost immediately he is completely broken; his burden is too great:

'Cursed be the day I was born! . . .
Why did I ever come out of the womb
   to see trouble and sorrow
   and to end my days in shame?'
               (Jer 20:14, 18)

At that point, however, the tone of the prophecy God gives gradually begins to change. Hope enters. There is the promise of the provision of faithful pastors, of a return from exile, of restoration after judgment, and of the coming of the Messiah himself (23:3–8). The preservation of a remnant is assured (24:4–7). The judgment of the oppressor, God's instrument of chastisement, is also sure (25:8–14). The note of hope becomes dominant (ch 30): God's purpose will be accomplished, and will culminate in the making of a new covenant. His people will be inwardly changed and live out the will of God (31:31–34).

Distinguishing the ladder from the treadmill

Elijah was on the ladder, but began to turn it into a treadmill and fell off. Jeremiah was, in God's providence, set on a hard ladder in the first place, and the Lord told him how hard it would be. But it *was* a ladder and its steepness almost broke him. At the point of breaking, when his hold on the Lord was almost gone, the Lord himself lifted him up and revealed to him where the ladder was leading. He continued to the end and reached the top. In both cases the Lord in his grace met each where he was and supplied the appropriate restoration.

We need to be able to distinguish between the two if we are to deal with them appropriately in ourselves or in others. My own problems, for instance, were of the Elijah type; I know others whose problems are of the Jeremiah variety and, indeed, some of my own present tendencies to depression and discouragement are of that type rather than the former and need to be dealt with in a different way.

God's answer to Jeremiah was simply to encourage him by giving him a vision of what his costly work was ultimately to lead to. To Elijah God said, almost in rebuke, 'What are you doing *here*, Elijah?'; implying that he should not have been there at all, even though the Lord restored him in grace and love.

Such discernment is very necessary today. A number of years ago I was acquainted with a medical missionary and his wife who were concerned to develop a novel kind of work in an area where it had not been tried before, though it had proved successful elsewhere. It required a considerable investment in equipment. On successive occasions equipment was sent out to the country concerned, only to be rendered useless and irreparable shortly after arrival by quite different, and completely unexpected, factors and disasters. Their reaction was, 'This is the devil trying to frustrate the work of God.' They persevered, to no effect.

The reaction of the minister of their home congregation was different. He asked, 'Is it not possible that in fact the *Lord* is saying that this is *not* the way forward?' Were they on a treadmill or a hard ladder? Their conviction that they were on a hard ladder brought them both near to breaking-point. In the event it proved to be a treadmill, and the results they hoped for were achieved as effectively and much more cheaply by other means.

How we need to pray for true Spirit-inspired discernment in these matters! It is so easy to become obsessively convinced that what is in fact a treadmill is a hard ladder which we have no alternative but to negotiate.

David

A different example is given by David. After his anointing by Samuel and his initial period in Saul's favour (1 Sam 16:1–23), David increasingly suffers through Saul's jealousy of his accomplishments (1 Sam 18:6–9) and is forced to become an outlaw (1 Sam 21:1–10).

Despite respecting Saul's life on two occasions, because he was God's anointed king, he becomes increasingly disillusioned and starts to doubt whether God really will perform the promise implied in his own anointing. He has had so many narrow escapes that he becomes convinced that, sooner or later, Saul will get him. So, for sixteen months, he and his men throw in their lot with the Philistines against Saul and the people of Israel. While there he wreaks havoc among the Philistines in their remoter strongholds, lying to his Philistine hosts so that he would not be detected, and ruthlessly destroying all who might have revealed the truth (1 Sam 27:7–11). God has to ensure that David is sent back to his proper place of service until God's time for him to take up the kingship has come (1 Sam 29:1–31:13).

God had given David, as a young man, a vision of his future role in God's plans. When that proved to involve the climbing of a hard ladder, David tried to opt out. As he became more and more discouraged and depressed, he came to the point where he left the people of God and effectively sided with the enemy.

If challenged, no doubt he would have pointed out that he was killing large numbers of the enemy. But it involved deceit and lying, all with the frantic enthusiasm that is born of doing the work of God in our own way and our own strength. Rats on a treadmill can be very active and enthusiastic. But as with the rats, all the enthusiasm, effort and superficial numerical success does nothing to further the real purpose. It was only when David returned to the ladder that God's purpose for him could be accomplished.

It is in David's psalms that his character can most clearly be discerned. There is little doubt that, underneath all his ability as a soldier, king and leader, he was deeply sensitive, prone to extremes of elation and despair, feeling deeply the whole gamut of human emotions, and being profoundly conscious of both the excellence of righteousness and the heinousness of sin.

He was capable of supreme confidence in God, of considerable compassion, and yet also of cold ruthlessness – shown in the murder of Uriah and the massacres of the

Philistine communities. Yet Psalm 51 shows the agony of his guilt and the pain of his repentance. Few of the psalms he wrote can be directly related to the period with which we are concerned – perhaps Psalms 34, 52, 54, 56, 142 and one or two others – but the general picture of him presented to us by the scriptures leaves little doubt that he must have possessed a personality prone to depression.

His flight to Achish in Gath (1 Sam 27:1–7) was surely a depressive reaction. Like Elijah, he sought refuge from himself by running away from the circumstances in which he was. Too many Christians do the same. The ladder becomes a little hard, and so they try to find another one, and often the devil provides a convenient treadmill in an easily accessible position – an inviting prospect which leads nowhere.

Many Christians who opt for a change of this kind do so long before they are as desperate as David was, and with less reason for desperation. Some Christians spend their lives looking for the ideal church to provide them with a congenial ladder. Others leave one church and join another for quite inadequate reasons.

Still others effectively opt out by giving all their effort to extra- and para-church organizations. There are far more now than there ever have been and, no doubt, some are fully justifiable. Others, in my view, are not, and some are positive snares for unwary saints. Such organizations can be seen by discouraged and depressed Christians as an exciting alternative to the rather dull ladder which God has set up for them in their local church.

Living within the visible body

Membership of the body of Christ is more than an activity in which to engage. It means belonging to a community which, if it is to display the love of Jesus, will inevitably involve learning how to get on with, indeed to *love*, a disparate group of people of different ages, abilities, social backgrounds, sexes, interests, gifts and personalities. In other words, attending the local church but being active and involved in extra-church organizations, can be a cop-out. It avoids facing the problems of creating the community which alone can bear a full witness to Jesus Christ in the world, and within which the full saving and healing work of God can proceed.

The question we all have to ask before God is simple: 'Am I on a ladder which the Lord has put me on; or on another (which is in fact a treadmill) which I have chosen for myself?' In other words 'Am I in the place where God wants me to be serving him, even if it is hard, unrewarding and unspectacular? Or have I taken an easy option by working largely or completely outside the local church for reasons of personal preference rather than at the call of God?'

David's place in the purpose of God was among the people of God, however faithless and poorly led they seemed to him to be, and however much he knew in his own heart that sooner or later he was to be their leader. All his active and enthusiastic slaying of their enemies was useless because it was done in his own strength and at his own decision, not at the leading of God.

Certainly the Israelites were only the visible embodiment of God's universal purpose; those who were truly loyal to him were not necessarily the physical descendants of Abraham. But that did not mean that the nation was of no importance to God as a nation. The proper place of service for God's servants was *within* that identifiable entity, not outside it. Likewise with the relations between the visible and the invisible church today. The New Testament was written to *visible* churches, not to some indefinable subset within them.

Modern evangelicalism has to a significant degree neglected the importance of the visible church. Since the invisible church is known only to God, the whole concentration of energy has therefore been upon the individual Christian in his salvation, devotion and service. However, the Christian as an individual is born again *into the body* of Christ, which is his church. That body is certainly not precisely definable by any man in terms of the individuals who compose it, for only God sees the body of the bride of Christ naked in her absolute beauty. The visible church is the clothes she wears in this present evil world, however ill-fitting, torn, ragged and dirty they may sometimes be. But the bride is certainly inside the clothes and not outside them.

The lesson we need to learn is that individual Christians must live within the visible church as a vital part of the body of Christ. Even those who *are* called to work in extra-church Christian activities need deep roots in the visible, local church. As soon as those activities become an attempt to escape from the inevitable stresses and strains within the fellowship, we must beware. Extra-church activities cannot provide the corporate nurture and care which all Christian life needs if it is to grow to a healthy and useful maturity.

Other Old Testament examples

Elijah, Jeremiah and David show us that our problems today are not new. Other Old Testament characters provide helpful examples to study.

Nehemiah learnt the wisdom of setting the secular and material firmly in a spiritual context (see, for example, Neh 1:1–11; 2:4–9)

Abraham, Jacob and Rebekah learnt the folly of trying to work out God's purposes for them in their own way (Gen 16:1–16; 27:1–28:9).

Moses learnt the dangers of taking on too much and of not being prepared to delegate (Exod 18:5–26). He also demonstrates that God can make a major leader, a meek servant and a friend out of a man who displays many weaknesses of personality and character (compare Exod 3:1–4:13, especially 4:10–13, and Deut 32:48–52, with Deut 34:10–12).

Saul, on the other hand, began to rely on his own considerable strength, wisdom and ability, thus turning the ladder into a treadmill. (See 1 Sam 9–31.) He was a man of great natural gifts, but did not consecrate them to God for use in his way. Rejected by God as the leader of his people, he developed a mental illness, becoming moody and insecure, displaying symptoms of recurrent depression and developing paranoia. What the illness was we can only surmise, but the point is simple: his great gifts were not given back to God to use in his way, for his purposes. The root cause of *his* depression was indeed spiritual but, as we have seen from other examples, not all such mental disturbance is at root spiritual failure.

Paul wrote of the Old Testament, 'these things occurred as examples to keep us from setting our hearts on evil things as they did . . . These things happened to them as examples and were written down as warnings for us, on whom the fulfilment of the ages has come' (1 Cor 10:6,11).

11
Under pressure in the New Testament

Peter

In the New Testament, we rely more on implication than incident for our examples. Consider Peter, the strong-minded, impulsive activist. The Lord chose him as an apostle, saw him as a leader among the select band of twelve, recognized his natural gifts, but also saw his weakness and self-confidence.

Very often in the gospel story Peter's words and actions imply, as he looks at his fellow disciples, 'I'm not like them . . . I'm stronger, more loyal, more faithful, altogether more useful to you, Lord.' It is all there in a nutshell in his outburst of protested devotion at the Last Supper, 'Even if all fall away on account of you, I never will . . . Even if I have to die with you, I will never disown you . . .

Lord, I am ready to go with you to prison and to death'
(Matt 26:33,35; Luke 22:33). In Gethsemane he keeps to
his resolve, draws his sword and attacks one of the arresting
party – and is rebuked by the Lord for doing so.

Peter was on the treadmill of trying to serve his Lord
according to his own knowledge and understanding, his
own vision and perceptions. Before he could be used in the
purpose of God, he had to be broken and to learn true
dependence and simple obedience. A few hours after he
had spoken so strongly of his faithfulness he was a defeated,
sobbing wreck of a man. Even after Jesus' resurrection the
defeat and depression were still present. When the disciples
returned to Galilee to wait for the Lord, there was a hint
of desperation in Peter's statement, 'I'm going out to fish'
(John 21:3). His self-esteem was shattered, his hope still
very insecure, his leadership aspirations shown for the sham
they were, and his understanding of the purpose of God
still vague and uncertain. So he turned back to what he
knew he could do – fish. And even that failed.

Peter had come to know through the bitterest experience
that in himself he had no strength to do the work of God;
he could not withstand the pressure and stress. At that
point of defeat and brokenness his Lord met him. Jesus
began to teach him the way of effective service. The new
Peter of Pentecost began to grow, ready to be used by the
Spirit of God to found the church by the gospel of the risen
Christ. God's use of Peter at Pentecost would have been
impossible without the death and resurrection of Peter's
personality through his denial, his brokenness, his defeat
and depression. God had to create a Peter he could use,
who had sacrificed his own claim to use his gifts and talents
as he thought best. They were then utterly at his Lord's
disposal.

So, from the experience of Peter, we can learn that God
has a purpose in our pain and defeat; it is not an end in
itself, it is a means to an end. If we break under the pressure
of that defeat, God can bring us through to a frame of mind
and heart which is much more usable by him than that

which preceded breaking-point. He can use our falling off the treadmill to plant our feet on an even more glorious ladder – if we let him.

Paul

What of the other great apostle, Paul, the founder of so many Gentile churches, to whose ministry we ultimately owe our own conversion? He needed to be broken and restored in a different way from Peter.

There is little in his writings or the record of his ministry to warrant the conclusion that he ever suffered from any kind of clinical depression, but a great deal which shows the depth of feeling and almost unbearable concern involved in his ministry to the churches he and others had founded. His goal was that they should be established in the truth of the gospel, grow into maturity of faith and love, and be convincing witnesses to the power of Christ's love. As it moulded the very different groups of people, and the individuals of which they were composed, into coherent, concerned, compassionate, caring, worshipping communities, the power of that love would be seen.

To the church at Corinth, he wrote:

'Praise be to the God and Father of our Lord Jesus Christ, the Father of compassion and the God of all comfort, who comforts us in all our troubles, so that we can comfort those in any trouble with the comfort we ourselves have received from God. *For just as the sufferings of Christ flow over into our lives, so also through Christ our comfort overflows. If we are distressed, it is for your comfort and salvation; if we are comforted, it is for your comfort, which produces in you patient endurance of the same sufferings we suffer.'*   (2 Cor 1:3–6, italics mine)

The subsequent verses indicate that Paul's thoughts may have been largely on physical persecution and bodily pain;

but he cannot be excluding mental and psychological anguish. There is a psychological as well as a spiritual cost to all real Christian service, and it is difficult to separate the two.

Paul, being a greater servant than most, undoubtedly also suffered more acutely than most. There can be no real Christian service without cost. This is different from the pressure and stress brought on by driving ourselves in essentially self-centred service. It is rooted in the cosmic conflict between good and evil in which we are inevitably involved if we seek to go God's way rather than that of the prince of this world.

The victory *was* finally won for God by the 'proper man', as Luther put it, Jesus Christ, on the cross, and proved by his resurrection and ascension. We, as servants of that Lord, are inextricably caught up in the working out of that victory in our daily lives, and supremely so in our efforts to make the whole of our lives the vehicle of God's grace. *That* is the battle, and battles cost. If we are called by God to Christian leadership then the cost can be great; we are in the forefront of the battle, for no truly faithful Christian leader attempts to lead from behind. He follows his Lord to the front line.

When, earlier in my life, I wanted to go forward for the ordained ministry of the church, my father said to me, 'Son, you take that road only when the Lord has closed all the others.' Now that God has given me that vocation, nearly forty years later, I understand more clearly than ever before the wisdom of that advice.

Since the mental suffering of the apostle Paul was the direct result of the ministry which God had given him, he could draw fully on God's grace to sustain him and could truthfully say:

'In all these things we are more than conquerors through him who loved us. For I am convinced that neither death nor life, neither angels nor demons, neither the present nor the future, nor any powers, neither height nor depth,

nor anything else in all creation, will be able to separate us from the love of God that is in Christ Jesus our Lord.'
(Rom 8:37–39)

Paul was not talking abstract theology; he was speaking from personal and sometimes bitter experience. Consider the apostle's ministry. He moved from city to city preaching and teaching; small groups of believers were left behind in each place he visited. Frequently he was forced to move on long before he would have wished, leaving behind a church poorly instructed in the faith, and vulnerable to every stratagem of the evil one in his efforts to spoil and destroy the work of the Lord. How frustrated he must have felt at times, perhaps wondering whether his work would last at all! So he was forced to write letters in order to correct error, to provide further instruction, to comfort and instruct the groups of believers which were the fruit of his evangelism. Those letters now form a large part of our New Testament. If Paul had not been forced into the position he was, the church, including us, would not have had the priceless treasure of the permanent teaching contained in those letters.

Remember too, that many of Paul's letters were written from prison. The apostle would not have chosen to be in prison, but had he been able to conduct an uninterrupted evangelistic mission he would have had no time to write those letters, to the loss of nearly twenty centuries of Christian history. Paul's practical trust in God was strong enough to enable him to put to eternal use every experience through which the Lord led him. His whole aim was to please his Lord, and not to question his leading. He built a well-constructed superstructure on the foundation which had been laid – God's revelation of himself through the scriptures of the Old Testament, and his personal knowledge of and total commitment to Jesus Christ. That commitment cost in many other ways as well (2 Cor 11:23–29).

We are called to similar commitment (2 Cor 6:1–10). Our main safeguard against coming to breaking-point is the same as that of the apostle – to build a well-constructed faith on the solid foundation available. Then we shall be happy to let the Lord use us for his purposes, even if we consider that he is not using us in the way we would think the best and most effective. God sees long-term; our longest view is short in his terms. Obedience and self-discipline must become our way of life.

We must, more and more, make scripture a part of our very make-up, individually and corporately. Regular habits of prayer and praise must be developed, at both the personal and the community levels. Regular and frequent corporate worship become the first priority. The sacraments too should be given their appropriate place in that worship as real means of grace. If we get this core right then our church and extra-church activities will fall into their proper places and the orientation of our whole lives will be actually and consciously towards God. We shall then become increasingly able to sustain the pressure and stress that is part of the battle because we shall be firmly and securely climbing the ladder of loving duty to God.

Jesus

A demanding calling

We are called to *follow* Jesus:

'Come to me, all you who are weary and burdened, and I will give you rest. Take my yoke upon you and learn from me, for I am gentle and humble in heart, and you will find rest for your souls. For my yoke is easy and my burden is light.'

(Matt 11:28–30)

Surely no words of scripture are more relevant for those who are under pressure. These are more than words of comfort, they ask us actually to *do* something: 'come . . . take upon you . . . learn'.

The picture of the *yoke* is significant, and important to our understanding of the invitation. It was a simple piece of wood with appropriately located vertical pegs which linked two oxen together so that they might perform various tasks – like ploughing or hauling a wagon – in partnership together. A good yoke of oxen was a pair of animals similar in size and strength who, when linked by a yoke, could perform such tasks together efficiently and effectively. An unmatched pair would not only be inefficient, but also a trial to one another and, by reason of that, ineffective. Furthermore, a well-constructed yoke would be properly fitted to the animals it was to be used by, so making their task of working together easier and less stressful and pressured; such was an 'easy' yoke.

The yoke also had a training function. A young ox would be yoked together with an older and more experienced animal. By working with him, the untrained one would learn the most effective way of performing the tasks set and how to respond to the signals and indications given by the farmer using the yoke. Hence the link between 'taking' the yoke, and 'learning' in Jesus' invitation. With a well-matched pair of oxen and a well-fitted yoke, even a large burden could be made to seem 'light', since the effectiveness of the effort expended would be maximized.

This background illuminates Jesus' words. He is not representing himself primarily as the farmer who determines the task, but as the fellow ox to whom he invites us to be yoked. The yoke to which he invites us is 'easy', that is, designed specifically for each individual who accepts the invitation. The purpose of the yoke is that we should *learn* from him, not primarily in an intellectual sense, but in a practical way, in constant obedience to his promptings through the yoke which links us to him.

The 'lightness' of the burden is not determined by its intrinsic size and character, but by the compatibility of the two persons involved. Thus the more we become like Jesus and the more closely we conform to his movements and guidance, the less heavy the burden will seem. He promises that the yoke will fit perfectly. Any chafing and unease will be the result of our deviating from his promptings, not because his demands are unreasonable or beyond our capacity to meet. We will not be tested beyond our ability. However, as we grow to maturity in a yoke with him, the demands will become inherently more difficult and demanding. For he offers us a rest which is not the stagnation of inactivity or the self-indulgence of lazy comfort; but the rest of healthy, effective work, supported by a partner of infinite strength and compassion, and interspersed with periods of true relaxation.

These words of Jesus sum up almost completely much of what has already been inferred from the biblical evidence about the causes and prevention of stress. His promise is to those who are weary and burdened. His offer is a new, alternative way of service – a rejection of the exhausting and futile treadmill, and an acceptance of the ladder to be climbed, while being securely yoked to him.

Jesus had no special advantages

We sometimes think that somehow Jesus had a great advantage over us in facing the problems and testings of life because he was God come in the flesh. This is simply not so, as the writer of the letter to the Hebrews makes plain:

' . . . it is not angels he helps, but Abraham's descendants. For this reason he had to be made like his brothers in every way . . . Because he himself suffered when he was tempted, he is able to help those who are being tempted. We do not have a high priest who is unable to sympathise with our weaknesses, but we have one who has been tempted in every way, just as we are – yet was without sin.' (Heb 2:16–18; 4:15)

More than that:

'During the days of Jesus' life on earth, he offered up prayers and petitions with loud cries and tears to the one who could save him from death, and he was heard because of his reverent submission. Although he was a son, he learned obedience from what he suffered.'

(Heb 5:7, 8)

Jesus was subjected to all the pressures and stresses, all the problems and testings, which we experience. In fact, much more! Being without a sinful heart to seduce him away from the pathway God had set before him, all his testings were directly from the devil himself. Jesus' battle was harder, not easier, than ours. His testing was far more severe than any of his people are called to bear, whether physical, psychological or spiritual. Like us, his victory had to be won through faith, by trust in and obedience to his Father.

The key to Jesus' victory was his ability to discern infallibly the will of God, not only generally, but also particularly. Outwardly his mission appeared to be a failure. Despite close contact with him over three years and profound teaching from him, his disciples failed to understand what his work was all about. At his death they were not nearly ready to follow through the work that he had begun. Yet he could say at the Last Supper that it was *good* that he should go away! His ministry could have lasted much longer, and common sense showed that it should. His disciples still needed him, and there were still thousands of people needing healing of body, mind and spirit. Yet on the cross he could cry in triumph, 'It is completed!' Although that clearly refers primarily to his work of redemption on the cross, it cannot exclude the work he did before his death. He had fulfilled the work that God gave him to do, completely, down to the last detail.

In our far humbler role in God's purposes we need to do the same. God does not call us to rush around trying to meet every need, supporting every cause that comes to our attention, and feeling that we have sinned when we fail to do so. The Lord calls us to fulfil *our* part in *his* total work; no more, no less. His will needs to be discerned by a mind fed on the scriptures and guided by the Holy Spirit. Jesus' life is of supreme significance to us as the perfect example of a life lived totally by faith in God, his Father.

He knew pressure and stress. He wept over the death of Lazarus and over the bitter hardness of heart of Jerusalem. He was watched, tested, taunted and hunted by Jewish religious leaders. In Gethsemane he perspired in an agony of apprehension, alone and forsaken by his friends. On the cross, when all his disciples had forsaken him and fled in fear, he knew the desolation of being abandoned by the Father whom he had loved and served perfectly throughout his life. Because he was bearing our sin and guilt he took on his lips the words of the most grim and desolate stanza of the psalms, 'My God, my God, why have *you* forsaken me?' David's Lord and God takes to himself the words of David, his human ancestor, uttered at one of the many times when he was in the depths of the most profound depression, and under extreme pressure and stress. He thus identifies himself wholly and completely with the hideous reality of human sin and with the deepest depression, as he is subjected to unendurable physical, mental and spiritual pressure.

However deserted, lost and crushed you may feel, your Lord knew worse, far worse. In no sense had he brought it on himself, as to some extent each one of us has. He bore it for you so that he might understand and truly sympathize with other broken, desolate souls. Jesus knows by his own experience exactly how you feel! Hold on to that, for he will bring you through by the same power and grace that brought him through to victory and glorious resurrection. How gracious and sympathetic is our Lord and Saviour! He is with us even when we exhaust ourselves on the treadmill, just as he is with us on the steepest and hardest ladder.

12
Practical actions

The practical actions which we now begin to look at are
really an outworking of the principles we have seen already.
There is no magic carpet to take us up the ladder without
climbing rung by rung. That means effort, action, decision
and hard thinking about the practicalities of the life of faith.
Certainly the Holy Spirit of God is intimately involved in
all this, but he does not act apart from our cooperation.
We must use our minds, and actually take steps to live a
certain kind of life.

The necessity of self-discipline

The first practical element is the absolute necessity for self-discipline. God is not going to do by an instant miracle what he intends to do through me. Nor is he going to provide me miraculously with what he intends me to work out for myself. He is not going to bypass the mind he has renewed for me by the regenerating power of his Spirit (Rom 12:2).

Priorities

Self-discipline must be exercised first in the use of time. Most of us need to look very carefully at our priorities afresh before the Lord, and have the courage to put things right where it is necessary to do so. If we try to meet all the demands on our time we will simply run out of it. So what should our priorities be? The order of importance which follows has been partly implied in what has already been written.

For those of us who are employed it is clear that our daily job must take up a large block of time. For those with clearly fixed hours, the amount of time is well-defined. Others, whose responsibilities can easily expand to fill all the time available, may have real problems over where to draw the line. In either case it is important to recognize God's calling. If God has called us to that work then he expects us to do it properly, and it takes priority over church *activities*. We need, however, to watch very carefully that our work never becomes important purely for itself rather than because it is done in service to God.

For mothers at home there is a glorious opportunity to turn the daily round that is often boring into an offering to the Lord. The influence for good on the children can be incalculable. There also, however, a watch is needed. A legitimate pride in the home can easily become selfish and express itself in a meticulousness which can tolerate nothing out of place and no hint of deterioration or dirt.

Those in 'full-time' Christian service in both church and

para-church organizations also need to watch their attitude to work. It too can become a god in itself, and we can then glory in the fact that we have a well-run parish, or well-organized church, or an efficient, economically run Society, rather than in the God whose work it is.

The only insurance against this is to put worship at the head of the list of our activities, the first priority on the time we have when our work is done. This includes personal, family and corporate worship. They are interconnected and they flow into one another. None should be neglected, but corporate worship is perhaps the key to getting our priorities right in the rest of our lives.

Corporate worship reminds us constantly that we are only part of the body of Christ. Our role in the church and in the world is only a part of the total purpose of God. We are inescapably dependent upon others and it is only in the company of the people of God that we make our personal pilgrimage up the ladder. Corporate worship embraces both our Sunday acts of worship and our midweek prayer and praise meetings.

Furthermore, I am convinced that part of that public worship each week should be the worship of the whole church – families together in church, with all the other members of the local congregation. This is an essential foundation for true family solidarity, and the one which makes its other expressions of solidarity holy and a glory to God.

Then time must be found to spend together as families and to engage in the Christian grace of hospitality, particularly towards the lonely, who are not by any means always old.

When these priorities have been settled, and only then, we can begin to look at activities and organizations both in the church and outside it and the contributions we might make to them. It may seem harsh and dogmatic to say so, but it may be that when activities take priority over opportunities for worship and prayer then they are, quite simply, *wrong* for us to engage in.

Finally, let it be said that our present patterns of services and midweek meetings for prayer and praise – morning service, evening service, and a prayer meeting and Bible study on Wednesday or Thursday – are not divine appointments, and that perhaps the time has come for a radical look at the way we use weekends and time our meetings. (There is further comment on this in the Appendix.)

It may seem strange that evangelism has been omitted from the list of activities. There are two reasons for this. First, the church is most effectively evangelistic by simply *being* herself. If she is a truly worshipping and praying community she will inevitably be a witness and challenge to the world outside, because the contrast will be so striking. Evangelistic *activity* will grow quite naturally out of that.

Then, second, the areas in which we seek to evangelize should grow naturally out of our daily lives – from our homes in the localities in which we live, and in our work in the offices, shops, factories, hospitals, schools and so on where we spend such a large proportion of our time. There again, the emphasis upon the quality of our life as children of God will be paramount in our witness, and the quality of our church life will also be vital. These in turn depend completely upon the quality, vitality and discipline of our worship – our response to the grace of God in our individual and corporate lives.

So we come back again to the primary importance of worship and prayer. Effective evangelism should be the inevitable outcome of the spiritual life of the body of Christ, not primarily a separate, organized activity undertaken sporadically or even regularly. It is in worship and prayer that God communicates his presence and refreshes, renews and revitalizes his church and her individual members. The sad thing is that while evangelism should be part of the climbing of the ladder, we have made it yet another separate treadmill. We have brought many to breaking-point by doing so.

Relaxation

We need to learn how to relax. This does not mean allocating large portions of our time to what is essentially selfish pleasure. Rather, it is teaching ourselves how to switch off.

This can be done in a number of ways. Some do it easily by engaging in an activity like music, walking or sport which diverts attention away from the ordinary activities of life with its pressures and stresses. Others of a more passive disposition may find that watching a film or play, either in a cinema or theatre or on the television, has the same result. Further, physical and mental relaxation are connected. Relaxation exercises can be learnt and practised. Although mastering the full relaxation of every muscle, as well as the mind, may be a slow process, it is eminently worthwhile.

Many Christians tend to consider relaxation of any deliberate kind a waste of time that ought to be used in the Lord's work. In my view this is a false economy. The work of the Lord done in the shorter available time may well be more effective and more thoroughly done than that crammed into every available moment. Without deliberate relaxation we are likely to come to breaking-point much more quickly, especially if we have a personality and general make-up which is liable to crack-up – and often we do not find that out until it actually happens!

Saying 'No'

A further virtue to be cultivated is the ability to say, 'No', politely of course! This is not as easy as it sounds, as many who have tried it have found. It is important because every additional commitment, whether continuing or a 'one-off', is an extra item of potential pressure and stress.

We are programmed with the ready 'Yes, I will be able to do it,' because we are flattered by being asked, or constrained by our sense of Christian duty, or anxious to be seen as active Christians, or think we know that, if we decline, a certain other person whom we consider far less fitted for the task will be asked. We may also be afraid that our keenness will be doubted if we say 'No'. Instead we must evaluate our capacities realistically. For most involved Christians, the taking on of a new, continuing responsibility will mean dropping another. Much depends of course upon the nature of the responsibilities and commitments; but at the very least the two commitments must be evaluated against each other. Simply to take on a fresh activity is inevitably to increase the pressure.

We need to see our lives in total if we are approached to take on something extra. It is useless to point out that if I do not do it then it will not get done, or it will be done less efficiently. The real question is, 'Does *God* want *me* to do this?' If he does then we must examine the rest of our commitments in life and decide which one of those God does *not* want done, and give it up. The Lord is not in the business of driving his servants to breaking-point.

With one-off engagements the problem is different, but such commitments can readily fill the diary. It is very easy to try to fit something into an already tight schedule in order to please or help someone. It may occasionally be justified, but again the crucial question relates to what *God* wants – and that also applies to secular and social invitations.

We need to so practise the presence of God that he is brought into these decisions as a habit of life. It is vital that we assess how much we can take on in a specified period of time, in the light of the priorities we have established and the regular commitments we have, and to pace our occasional commitments accordingly. When we reach our allocation for a particular period, we need to say, 'No. I'm sorry, but I am fully committed for that period.' The commitment possible in that period is *not* determined by the spaces available in the diary; it is controlled by the amount of work that I can take on without excessive strain in that period. There *ought* to be blank spaces in the diary – they will only be filled in the direst emergency. The commitment involves not only the duration of the meeting, but also the time we need for preparation. In addition, the preparation of our minds and hearts spiritually before God is a necessity when we are asked to minister the word of God. We must learn the art of saying 'No' graciously.

Support of marriage and family

In all this the blessings of a good wife or husband cannot be overestimated. Of course, some are called to celibacy for various reasons, as both our Lord and the apostle Paul make quite clear. If, however, God has called us to marriage, he intends us to work together.

By marriage a new unit for worship and service is created (see Gen 2:24, Matt 19:1–12, Eph 5:22–33). The husband or wife is both inside and outside the life of the other half of the unit. Each is in a unique position with respect to the other. On the one hand we need to observe our partner in order to detect signs of pressure and stress, and to keep a sensitive eye on the commitments undertaken. On the other, we must take seriously what our partner sees and communicates to us. We need to talk these things through regularly, and to work out our joint priorities, our relaxations, our allocation of time. If we have children they too have to be considered and perhaps, as they grow, be brought into some of our discussions. Home should be the place where we can be ourselves, without restraint; but the building of such a home involves effort in cooperation with God's grace.

Within the marriage bond the physical relationship between the sexes has its part to play. A satisfying relationship here can be a significant bonus which can actually reduce and dissipate pressure and stress. On the other hand, an unsatisfactory physical relationship in marriage can exacerbate the pressures that stem from other sources. The physical dimension of the relationship is the sign and seal of the rest of the relationship which exists at less tangible levels. God intends that it should be used as such to the blessing of his children in their service of his kingdom together.

Decision-making and problem-solving

Problems and decisions need to be faced only once – when they occur. We tend to ask the question, 'What would I do if . . . ?' and so become anxious and worried. 'Do not worry about tomorrow, for tomorrow will worry about itself. Each day has enough trouble of its own' (Matt 6:34). Jesus' words may be taken as a command. The Lord expects us to face problems as and when they occur, deciding on a course of action according to an evaluation of the factors which we discern at that time, and our appreciation of the facts that are available to us. He does not hold us responsible for the facts we do not know, or the factors of which we are unaware. Although we need to consider the possible consequences of various courses of action, the Lord does not reveal to us a detailed plan of action extending into the remote future. Instead we are guided step by step, rung by rung, decision by decision. We know where we are going, but we do not know the details of the way; from our perspective it is still hidden but the next step is always clear. That is what living by faith means.

There is a further consequence of the rung by rung approach – we do not look back either, continually questioning the rightness of decisions made in the past. If they have been made before God, in honesty, according to the information available at the time, then they were *right* decisions and will fall into place in the purpose of God as rungs on the ladder.

Of course, in many instances we would have made a different decision if we had known *then* what we know *now*. The point is, we *didn't* know it. The rightness or wrongness of a decision depends only upon our openness before God when we made it, and our honesty in looking at all the options open at the time in the light of what we knew then. The paradox is that as we progress up the ladder we begin to see that even our wrong decisions are used by God to teach us and thus to help us up the ladder.

It sometimes seems that we have a wrong view of the way the Lord guides his children. His call is, 'Follow *me!*', and not, 'Follow the route marked out in detail on this map.' Discerning his guidance is not a complicated exercise in orienteering. It is simply doing what he says – following *him*.

I have lost count of the number of people – mostly young – who have come to me, perplexed, anxious, desperately earnest and sincere, and asked, 'How do I find out God's plan for my life?' The answer is simple. Take each step as it comes, and walk with Jesus. The plan will then be revealed as he leads you through it. The plan is revealed by our participating in it.

The image which such perplexed Christians seem to have in their minds is of a God up there, who, in his heavenly filing cabinet, has a detailed map for each Christian, which they must follow – or else . . . ! But just to make things difficult, he never allows any Christian actually to see the map for his life; all he does is to reveal a number of clues, some merely hints, others quite ambiguous, a few only relatively clear. The Christian is then left with the problem of using the clues to work out God's plan for his life, and following it. If he succeeds then all is well. If he doesn't, he is condemned to wander in the dark until he discovers the all-important clue which will put him back on the right road. Such assumptions are devilishly wrong. The Lord is only too willing to guide – but in *his* way, which demands as its only precondition that we are willing to follow *wherever* he leads.

Counselling people with problems of guidance often reveals that the *real* problem is that they are *not* willing. They have reservations about some, often only one, of the open options; or there is one which they prefer to the others. What they are really asking is that God should lead them in the way they want to go. Such attitudes are often buried deep, and have to be brought into the open before the real way becomes clear. The rule is: step by step, rung by rung. My testimony is that it works; and it is the testimony of many other Christians.

The blessings of a balanced lifestyle

The third set of practical conditions which minimize the likelihood of reaching breaking-point relates to lifestyle. They can be summarized by the words *balanced living*, and its requirements are all very practical, almost mundane.

Sensible eating

This implies not simply the avoidance of gluttony. It means the adoption of a sensible diet – not difficult to devise with the information available today. Most important, however, is the need to make time to eat with some leisure. Rushed meals and snatched snacks do no one any good.

In relation to this, how considerate are you of your church leaders? Do you tend to phone them at meal times, making demands on their time which curtails that available for relaxed eating? Leaders, ministers and others can also learn the art of saying politely, but firmly, 'Is your request really urgent, or can it wait until I have finished my meal? May I phone you back in a half-hour, or at some other convenient time?'

Social obligations

Our social obligations also need to be sensibly balanced.

Not least is the question of responsibility to in-laws and parents when the new family unit develops and marriage grows. This has already been mentioned as a significant source of pressure and stress. It has to be faced as such, but will not solve itself.

If the relatives concerned are Christians, the problem has to be worked out in Christian honesty and frankness between the family and the relations. The biblical pattern is clear: children have to leave the parental home and be united in the foundation of a new home and family (Gen

2:24). The separation has to be real and complete, and it places an obligation on *both* families. On the one hand the new couple are to *be united* by God into a new unit for his service. To do this they have to *leave* their respective parental homes and to break that link (though, of course, many responsibilities still remain).

On the other hand the parents must *give up* their respective children to the new unit which God has created. How hard Christian parents find it to do this! There must be no interference, no unreasonable social demands, no moral blackmail, no unasked-for advice, no veiled or open critical comment – however strongly we feel about particular issues and decisions. Yet Christian parents whose children have left the family home must always be there in the background with prayerful and loving support. This forms an almost impossible balance to achieve, and can only be done by the actively and constantly appropriated grace of God.

Children have obligations too. It is easy to make quite unreasonable demands of parents, especially when they become grandparents. They are not there to enable parents to lead the kind of life they did before the children were born – whether in maintaining 'worldly' or 'Christian' activities. That is not to say that grandparents may not have such a ministry; but the birth of children constitutes such a major change in the family unit that reappraisal of the whole pattern of life needs to be undertaken before God at that time. It may be that such reassessment of priorities will involve giving up some Christian activities in order to fulfil the family responsibilities that God lays upon parents. It does not follow that willing grandparents – especially grandmothers – are there to keep things going as they were before. Grandparents may have their holy calling in the church too!

With non-Christian grandparents the problems are different. Christian parents will want to give priority to the bringing up of their children in the faith, using Sunday especially for worship and teaching. But Sunday may well be the day when grandparents expect to see their families. Conflict and tension then arises. It is partly the result of our modern, mobile society. Not so long ago grandparents generally lived close at hand and could expect to see their grandchildren frequently, at times other than Sunday. If they *were* distant, visits would be special occasions. Mobility has made day and afternoon visits possible over much greater distances – at a cost in time, which so often has to be paid on a Sunday. Christians confronted with such a dilemma will want to keep Sunday different and make worship the priority. At the same time they may be afraid that denying the regular weekly visit to the grandparents will make them antagonistic to the claims of Jesus Christ and obstruct their coming to him, which is the deep desire of the Christian couple.

Two comments may perhaps help a little.

First, the conversion of the grandparents will be a work of God if it is to take place at all; our part is simply obedience to the word of God. Second, the most potent and powerful thing we can do is to pray for them, backing up our prayers by a life of faithfulness to God and loving consideration to them in their real needs. God is faithful to his promises and rewards our *faithfulness to him*, not our attempts to convert our relatives – whether by pandering to what are essentially selfish demands, or by incessantly preaching at them.

The same rule may also be applied to Christian children living with non-Christian parents, to relationships at work, and to the social obligations entailed by the nature of our employment. In essence it is the old cliché; we have to earn the right to speak. Earning that right is not brought about by pandering to unreasonable demands, but by working out in our lives the obedience of love which God asks of us – to him first, and then, as an inevitable consequence, to those close to us in human kinship or in social relation.

There are, in this whole area of our social and personal relationships, potential tensions that need to be dealt with in a biblical and loving way – another area in which the treadmill must be turned into a ladder, not only for ourselves but for others.

Material goods

We live in a society in which many pressures encourage us to equate happiness and contentment with the actual possession of material goods. We see, perhaps quite subconsciously, a certain level of housing, of furnishings, of transport, and of material goods in general, as necessary to our social and occupational standing.

As the expectations and standards of our fellows grow, so ours grow with them, and we are caught on another treadmill. The pressures on us are increased when they are brought to bear on our children, particularly at school, by the aspirations and material possessions of their contemporaries. At the very least, the unthinking acceptance of these pressures means that if our financial circumstances improve, we automatically spend our larger pay packet on things we couldn't afford before, or on an increased mortgage, when perhaps God intends that it should be devoted to the work of his church or to the needs of others.

Earning an increasing salary and a growing income is not a sin, but the way we spend it – or keep it – can be. We are not required to adopt a life of enforced and artificial poverty. I do suggest, however, that we should assess our expenditure in terms of what we can justify before God as needs; and not in terms of what we require in order to keep up with our contemporaries. The pressure to acquire is a treadmill, not a ladder.

Further complications can arise from this way of thinking. For example, a newly married couple decide to delay having children until they have established a comfortable home. This is clearly not wrong it itself. But suppose that in order to acquire a house which they think suitable, or equipment that they think vital, they take out a mortgage or a loan and involve themselves in debts which can only be met by their both working. Then a child arrives. The wife takes maternity leave and then returns to full-time work. The child is left in the care of a child-minder. Sometimes the arrangement works; but, apart from the question of whether Christian parental responsibility admits such a solution (as well it may if the person looking after the child is a loving Christian herself), what happens when the child is ill, or if the child is born handicapped in some way? The tension already created by the stretching of the child-parent bond may be brought to an unbearable level. Stress and pressure will again take their toll. It is then too late to backtrack without considerable difficulty and anxiety.

It is unfortunate that in our society today it is often economically necessary that both parents work – though I am not saying that it is wrong or even undesirable for both to be earning. But some of the problems which may arise will produce extra pressure and stress. These might be avoided if we adopted a more biblical approach to possessions and standards of living. Many of us need to engage in an honest and radical assessment of the pressures to which we have subjected ourselves over the course of the years. Then, by examining each source to identify those which are unnecessary, we can begin to reduce the pressure by cutting them out.

Medical care

Finally, there is the very practical step we can take of ensuring that we have regular medical care.

Again, a balance is needed. On the one hand we must avoid a neurotic preoccupation with our health and possible illness, treating every minor ache, pain or abnormality as though it presaged some fatal ailment. On the other, we need to avoid the carefree dismissal of symptoms – particularly the initial indications of developing pressure and stress, like irritability and impatience, indigestion through rushed meals, and so on.

The general practice with which my wife and I are registered, runs a clinic where those who are fit and well can have regular checks to assess their health, physical and mental. Many practices run similar clinics and we should use them. We need to be aware of the initial signs warning us that pressure is mounting up and to watch out for them in ourselves. We need to seek expert advice if we suspect that we are under excess pressure.

Learning to share

Close friends or relatives can usually be our best symptom-watchers. The development of close relationships in various areas of our lives is vital.

First, in the family. The marriage relationship and its importance have already been considered, but as children grow up and then leave to make their own lives, new relationships are possible which can be of mutual benefit and deepen as the years go on.

Relationships have to be based on a sound foundation, and have to be built carefully by mutual trust, honesty and love into reliable structures which can take the strain of sharing with and caring for each other. We have the foundation in our shared faith in the Lord, and how happy the human family that shares such a base! But deep relationships do not just happen, nor are they spontaneously created by the Holy Spirit in a single act of grace. They have to *grow*. They have to be nurtured – spiritually, socially and personally. Some Christian families have worked hard to create such quality relationships, built through worship, prayer, social activity, trust and honesty. Unfortunately not all Christian families are like that – but they can and should be.

For many Christians, however, from non-Christian homes or from Christian homes which do not yet approach God's ideal, the principal friendships will be developed within the local church community. The friends we need are not only of our own age, of similar social class, of the same profession or occupations, though all can be helpful. It is important to break across such social and age barriers and to avoid forming cliques. It is sad that the way we organize our churches often fosters the development of such spiritual ghettoes. I recall a Parochial Church Council at its day conference bitterly complaining that the congregation was divided into all sorts of groups which hardly ever mixed with one another. All sorts of solutions were proposed, mostly social events. The discussion was eventually silenced by one member, who said, 'What else can we expect when we organize the church on that basis?' That is so true of many churches. Their very organizational structure inhibits, and often completely strangles, any possibility of the growth of deep friendships between individuals in such different groups.

We also need to develop friendships with other Christians outside our own congregation – in other churches, in groups based on common professional and occupational interests, and with others who are subjected to similar kinds of pressure. There we shall find a sympathetic Christian understanding of those pressures which are the result of our own pattern of life.

We should also cultivate relationships with those who do not share our faith but who do share our interests and problems. One of the greatest bulwarks against breakdown is to have a wide circle of trustworthy friends to whom we can talk with reasonable freedom, on a basis of mutual trust. Naturally our relationships with those who are Christian will be at a deeper level, but let us not therefore despise the real friendship we can enjoy with those who are not. They are not to be seen as potential converts to be preached at but as people who can genuinely help us. We must be prepared to receive as well as give in such a relationship, for such friends may be wooed into the kingdom only on the basis of mutual respect and trust. None the less we need our Christian friends more.

Indeed, I am convinced that we need more than this. My High Church and Anglo-Catholic friends speak of the need for a 'spiritual director' to whom they can go for regular guidance in their Christian pilgrimage; someone to whom they confide their deepest needs, failures and sins, as well as seeking guidance and help in decisions and problems.

I am sure we all need such a friend, counsellor and guide. Some would say that someone of the same sex as the one directed is desirable, even necessary. I would say that is relatively unimportant and that qualities of character are far more significant. The director or special friend will be a mature Christian who has faced and solved problems, with a wealth of experience, and an evident store of wisdom and biblical understanding. It is therefore unlikely that the director will be young, though age in itself is no qualification. Above all the person will be *spiritual* – not ostentatiously pious, full of spiritual jargon and evangelical shibboleths, but with a whole life which is evidently orientated towards God and his will. Because the Lord is truly *known*, in the deepest sense, his (and 'his' includes 'her'!) personality will quietly radiate the realistic love of Jesus. He will command full respect and confidence, receive the deepest and most intimate confidences, burdens, sins, worries and revelations of the heart and life without condemnation and with no possibility of their being revealed beyond the one-to-one conversation. But he will share them with his Lord in prayer and communion. In return he will be fully honest and frank in that love which comes from Christ alone, even if what he has to say or advise hurts deeply, and makes the utmost demands on my faith, love and sacrificial discipline. To say or advise that which hurts will cost him as much as it costs me, but the relationship will show the kind of love described in 1 Corinthians 13:4–8. It is 'patient . . . kind . . . does not envy . . . does not boast . . . is not proud . . . is not rude . . . is not self-seeking . . . is not easily angered . . . keeps no record of wrongs . . . does not delight in evil but rejoices with the truth . . . always protects, always trusts, always hopes, always perseveres . . . never fails.' A friendship like this is not only a defence against pressure and stress becoming intolerable, but also provides healing if, despite all, breaking-point is reached.

Some may say that a living relationship with Jesus is all

that is needed; he is the friend that sticks closer than a brother. That is true; but just as he had to become man to be our friend, so his word has to become flesh in us in order that he may be *shown* to others. However real and intimate our times with the Lord are, we are still members of one another; we still need one another. Horizontal relationships constitute the very stuff of daily living. God does not leave us to climb the ladder alone and unaided. We climb it together, helping, supporting and loving one another.

The myth of indispensability

One last practical point remains to be made, one of basic significance. We need to explode the myth of our own indispensability. We like to think that we are indispensable at work, in the church, in the family. We might be *missed* if we were to die tomorrow, but the work would not stop. God's church would carry on; even the family would cope in due course.

To consider ourselves as indispensable is pure pride. In the context of our lives we are important only so long as we have our place in the purpose of God on this earth. When our role is fulfilled he will take us to our reward at precisely the right time; not a minute too soon and not a minute too late. Our indispensability is his decision not ours. The time when we reach the last rung of our particular ladder and step into glory will be determined by him and not by us.

The French word for a staircase is *l'escalier* and, for a port of call on a voyage or flight, *l'escale*. I like the link. Each step on the ladder is a port of call on our way to the ultimate destination – the glorious presence of the Lord. Let us enjoy the ports of call, but never stay too long, and remember always the destination.

PART FIVE

Broken by the mill:

for those who reach breaking-point

13
Self-help for the broken

'Our nightmare started one Saturday evening when my
husband came home from work looking haggard and
drawn with an ashen face . . . He could not eat and his
eyes looked strange and vacant. An hour or so later he
broke down . . . To my surprise, he made no objection
to visiting the doctor and somehow we dragged through
an interminable Sunday. He was astonished when the
doctor pronounced him profoundly depressed and
refused to allow him to work. *So much for being indispensable – now he had to get off the treadmill* . . . My husband,
the man who did not believe in nervous breakdowns, was
having one . . .'

(*The Guardian*, 29 January 1986. Italics mine)

Each of us has a unique psychological and physiological
make-up, and some are much more susceptible to pressure
and stress than others. In addition, each of us has a unique
history, a personal development, a past life, from which we
cannot escape. The mistakes of the past cannot be undone,
even if we change our lifestyle now. We are prisoners of

our past, and the past has a habit of exacting its dues to the last penny.

As the extract from *The Guardian* shows, it is too often those who believe they can stand the pressure who in fact break down under it. None of us can afford to exclude the possibility that it might happen to us. So we must consider seriously what should be done for the broken and crushed.

In my role as a pastor I would be keeping a close watch on those who, having read through the previous sections, say to themselves, 'It doesn't really apply to me; I can take it.' If that is coupled with a reaction to this section which says, 'I can skip this; it couldn't happen to me,' then I would be doubly concerned.

So what can be done for the rats who do fall off the treadmill? In this and the next chapter we will look at two dimensions. First, in what ways can they help themselves? Second, what can the rest of us do to help them?

Those who fall off the mill often feel quite unable to do anything about their condition. Because that feeling is part of the condition itself, self-help will involve a determined fight against hang-ups, and a search for encouragements. A number of areas on which to focus that determination may be readily identified.

Seek and take professional advice

This needs to be both physical and psychiatric. Many general practitioners are well aware of the psychological problems and have a special interest in them. It is necessary, anyway, to be sure that there are no physical problems that need to be dealt with. He may be sufficiently competent to deal with psychological problems, or he may refer you to a consultant. The professional competence of the psychiatrist is more important than whether or not he is a Christian. *Take* the advice you are given. If relaxation sessions are suggested, then attend them and practise the prescribed exercises. Half an hour each day, especially if you are able to continue working during the depression, is time well spent, not wasted.

Then we need to fight the hang-up we all have about pills, and drug-dependency. Our fears on this subject have been fed by the media. Added to which is the guilt we feel at taking pills, on the grounds that Christians should be able to deal with their mental states without such aids. Most of us are prepared to take paracetamol to relieve pain. But we drive a wedge between mind and body, and identify soul or spirit with the mind, and so come to despise or fear the use of drugs to aid the recovery of our mental stability. Often these fears are fed by the attitude of Christians who have not yet suffered acute depression.

There are books on *spiritual* depression, which are, in their own field, masterpieces of spiritual diagnosis and treatment. But few have much to say about the clinical depression which concerns us here. There is a difference. Spiritual depression is a hazard of the ladder; clinical depression is a danger associated with the treadmill. Of course they cannot be finally and completely separated; but they need to be distinguished despite their interaction. Elijah and Jeremiah were in different categories, though no doubt there were elements of both kinds of depression in each.

So be prepared to take drugs under proper medical supervision for as long as is necessary – but let the doctor decide what 'necessary' means. It may be desirable to take them for a prolonged period. Indeed, a low dose taken regularly on a permanent basis may be necessary to effect permanent stability. If that is so, then do not regret it; thank God for the provision and the care which enables you to continue to serve him and go out to do what he wants.

Of course God may heal without these means, but his glory is not diminished if he chooses to use pills to effect the cure. The timing of healing is his choice also; he has the right to make us wait for his own higher purposes. If healing does not occur at the time when we think it should, the prolonged illness should not be attributed to lack of faith or spiritual deficiencies on the part of the patient.

What about more drastic treatments – electro-convulsive therapy, injections or deep narcosis, for example? No responsible psychiatrist will suggest these unless he is convinced that other courses of action have failed or are unlikely to work. Nevertheless, it is worthwhile investigating the possible side effects of such treatments, almost all of which are only temporary, so that if and when they occur we are aware of what is happening. Here again we need to be ready to seek and take professional advice. It is always a great help if a relative or friend can be with us at such consultations.

Finally, we need to be prepared to take complete rest from all commitments for a period; maybe, quite literally, to get away from it all. We can be so reluctant to admit that we have fallen off the mill that we frantically try to keep up appearances. Here again medical advice is essential. In many cases of low-level depression, appropriate drug therapy can enable us to continue to do our daily job; but we are not indispensable. Some cutting down of commitments in other directions is always advisable; overcommitment is often a major factor in bringing us to breaking-point anyway. In deep depression a complete break, even a period in hospital, is almost always necessary. Our needs here must be assessed professionally. Left to himself the patient is liable to fall into one of two pits: either to try frantically to keep on as though nothing has happened, or to descend into deep withdrawal and attempt absolutely nothing.

Resist feelings of failure and guilt

Depressed Christians too often see themselves as defeated and useless failures. This can engender deep feelings of guilt, and exacerbate the whole condition. Tragically, such feelings are all too often reinforced by the words, actions and attitudes of other Christians. Guilt feelings do not necessarily reflect the existence of real guilt, but even if they do, that guilt is covered by the blood of Christ and is no longer held to our charge. His atoning death is an objective fact which is true quite independently of any *feelings* of guilt that I may have.

In a state of clinical depression there is an inbuilt tendency to *nurture* feelings of guilt, defeat and failure. These have to be resisted. From defeat and failure God can and will build something far more glorious and useful to himself and his purposes. It may be that breakdown is God's way of bringing us back to these fundamentals – his way of showing us the strength of our faith in him, which holds on despite all. Depression, and the feelings that go with it, can therefore be a witness *in themselves* to the grace of God, even while we are still going through it.

We need to try to engage in activities which we *can* cope with. Those of us whose work makes many demands on the intellect, may find manual tasks therapeutic. Even they will involve real effort though, so it is always a help to have someone who will encourage us to attempt things, and even work with us. Walking can also help, again in company if possible. What is best for us therapeutically will, however, depend upon the way in which breaking-point has come. Again we must be guided here by our medical adviser, especially if there are genuine organic damage points associated with our breakdown.

Help can also come from trying occupations which we once enjoyed but have long since given up under the pressure of time. Long-neglected hobbies can be revived and new ones tried. I wrote poetry of a kind (and still do) and found deep solace in music. We are all different, and we need to try to find activities which prevent us from sitting around completely inactive, dwelling on our sad state. Stress and depression should never be treated as though they were minor upsets to the system; they are traumas of a very profound kind, and those who have been through them are never the same again. Even modest tasks are desperately hard for the chronically depressed because, when we come to breaking-point and collapse off the tread-mill, we are always well and truly broken.

These practical steps may seem almost laughably simple and superficial to those who have never experienced depression of this kind; to anyone who is clinically depressed they seem almost insuperable barriers. Even attempting a jigsaw puzzle, or playing a game of Happy Families can demand an effort comparable to trying to play a game of chess with a Grand Master. To try them is, however, to relieve the despair and guilt just a fraction; and that is good and necessary. I well remember how much I was helped when, by a desperate effort of will, I had played just one indifferent set of tennis, and a medical friend who was with us said (when I had given up) 'That was good!' And for me, it was.

Determine to maintain a spiritual discipline

The last thing the chronically depressed person wants to do is to worship, to read the scriptures and to pray. When the effort is made it seems to yield little in spiritual comfort or produce any real change in the psychological condition. The discipline must be maintained, however, and the effort be made, for it is through the word, worship and prayer that the Lord will eventually work healing. It was through desultory Bible study that the Lord gave me a word to hold on to, and the assurance of light at the end of the dark tunnel.

Such spiritual discipline is hard work. We have to nerve ourselves to do it, to screw up our courage and fight, however feebly. We must remember that many of the greatest saints of God have been through the same and worse, coming out gloriously into new and richer service. So too, will the feeblest saint. At the time, however, all we have to hold on to is the promise of God. He is with us in 'the valley of the darkness that can be felt', even though we do not sense his presence, and it is only the sound of the tap of his staff on the road and the gentle touch of his rod which indicate his close walk with us. The din of the demons in the valley may almost drown out the steady tap, and the stench of their presence nearly obliterate any sense of his sweetness, but he has promised that he is there. To be sensitive to any token of the reality of that promise, we need to be reading his word, seeking him in worship and speaking to him in prayer. If we do not try to, however feebly, we deny ourselves the possibility of comfort and help.

Sooner or later all dark valleys open out on to the plain. God *will* bring us through to that outfall, however long and hard the road, not through the strength or weakness of our faith, but simply because he is that kind of God. We shall not be tested beyond that which we are able to bear and he knows what that limit is. We must tell ourselves this again and again – out loud, if necessary – until eventually we see the end of the trail, the darkness becomes less tangible, and light begins to break through.

It will now be clear why well-developed, caring relationships in the church fellowship are so important. They cannot be developed when the crisis strikes; they have to be there prior to its onset. This is also where a good marriage relationship tells. It is where I would see a spiritual director as being vital to the solution of the problem.

Having been developed before the depression or stress reactions strike, all these relationships have then to be kept up. That will depend to a great extent on the others, rather than the victim of depression, but even he can try to cooperate. It is very easy to succumb to separation from Christian fellowship, to avoid people, even those whom one holds most dear. They seem distant and unreal, they seem to become detached and unconcerned, and therefore not to matter any more. They, in general, have not changed; the feeling of distance and unreality is part of the depression. It is like living in a cloud of cotton wool which insulates against human contact. In such a state it is all too easy to opt out; that is dangerous, and must be resisted.

Never cease to believe that God will heal the depression

God may, in due time, provide sudden, even miraculous, healing. If he does, with or without a human agent, then rejoice and praise him for his grace and power. But whatever the time span and means he uses, the healing is always his healing. We ought not to engage in a frantic search for some spiritual healer to work the miracle; if God wishes to work that way, he will arrange the contact. Healing is, in my view, always best found in the local church, among the fellowship of Christians gathered together in prayer and worship. In its fullest sense it is a ministry of the church exercised as a whole, as the body of Christ.

In the healing of depression, the role of the spiritual director seems to me to be vital – in counsel, discernment and, if necessary, rebuke.

Healing can be hindered. I have argued that healing will come sooner or later, and I believe it will if it is desired unconditionally. Sometimes we impose conditions – perhaps hardly realizing it. Because our conditions are not met and we are not healed, we can become bitter, which further hinders our healing. Some, for example, find that their depression brings them attention which they have been desperately wanting. So they subconsciously impose a condition: they want to be free of the depression on condition that the attention from others is not lost. Other illnesses can of course be similarly used. The Lord may then not heal the depression because a deeper healing is required, to which the depression points. This can be discerned by a competent and loving spiritual director.

It grieves me to see individuals in the evening of their life in whom such roots of bitterness have grown – in relation to children who have left home, to brothers and sisters to whom they could have been so close, to friends who would otherwise have supported them. How much easier it would have been if they had been properly counselled by a competent spiritual adviser many years ago.

I am speaking of Christians, and perhaps for them the inevitable healing will be the ultimate one – death and passing into the presence of the Lord. Apart from the sacrificial caring of the local church and its members, they have condemned themselves to a lonely and disgruntled old age of fluctuating depression and self-pity. That is sad, and a warning to those of us who are younger. But wise counsel, prayer and a willingness to let go can still work wonders. Nevertheless, I know far more older people who are the exact opposite, who enjoy the love and care of many, and who give so much to those who help. They are not depressed even though they may be suffering severe physical disabilities of various kinds. They are near the top of the ladder; the former group is hanging on to a lower rung, refusing to loose their grip on that which holds them back.

Do not feel guilty about being angry with God

To some this will seem strange; to others dangerous; to yet others it will seem positively sinful!

Depression is a kind of bereavement; indeed it is a kind of loss of self, a deprivation of identity. The chronic depressive sees no point in his continuing to live; and that is true even if there is no attempt at suicide. Many who are depressed become, as I did, careless of their own safety in the normal course of life, thinking that it no longer matters whether they live or die.

In bereavement, anger against God is a common reaction. It is often a release of grief, and helpful in overcoming the deep deprivation of losing a loved companion and friend. So with depression.

158

But is it not wrong to be angry with God? God knows our make-up, and remembers our weakness (Ps 103:14). What is his reaction to our weakness and our anger? It is compassion:

'As a father has compassion on his children,
so the Lord has compassion on those who fear him.'

(Ps 103:13)

His *knowledge* of us is the basis of his compassion.

Job became angry with God over two things: what he saw as the unfair treatment he had received, and the fact that God would not listen to him or give him an answer. His words in Job 27–31, are those of a deeply angry man. Yet God does not reprimand him for his anger, only for his failure to appreciate the greatness and glory and care of God (Job 38–41).

Jeremiah showed anger when he cursed the day he was born, and not only anger but resentment at the lot which had fallen to him (Jer 20:7–9,14–18). Yet the Lord does not charge his servant with sin.

The New Testament exhortation in which Paul quotes from Psalm 4:4, implies that anger is something to be got out of the system:

' "In your anger do not sin": Do not let the sun go down while you are still angry.'

(Eph 4:26)

Of course, as Paul uses it, this refers to relationships within the Christian fellowship, but in our extremity of depression and despair the Lord understands our feelings of anger and absorbs them into himself. He can take it, not because they do not matter, but because they do, to us and to him. For anger against him is at least a recognition that he is there and has a part in the pain and desperation of the situation in which we are. His identification with us is shown supremely in the cross, and the triumph of his resurrection guarantees his ability to deal with it. That recognition is itself a step towards recovery; it should not be allowed to induce the guilt which would constitute a step backwards.

What has been said of anger applies to all the other feelings which plague us in depression. We must be open to God and not repress them before him, however ashamed of them we may be. He knows that they are there anyway, so why try to push them into the background and pretend that they are not there? Offer them to the Lord, direct them at him, and let him take care of them. Furthermore, if we have close Christian friends, and/or a suitable spiritual director, then we can open our anger, resentment, frustration, doubt, indeed all our abject misery, to them as well.

Being open to God in this way is one of the things that 'walking in the light' means (1 John 1:5–7). If we have made it a habit of life before we reach breaking-point it will be all the easier to practise it in the depths of depression. Do we share the deepest secrets of our hearts with him? Not only the ones we think he would like, but also those things of which we are deeply ashamed and which we could not share with anyone else? John links walking in the light with the confession of sin (1 John 1:8–10). Our admitting to these secrets by sharing them openly with the Lord, is the way in which we are released from them and the guilt and stress they bring with them.

Believe that the breakdown will, in the end, produce true good

This is perhaps the hardest thing of all. In the depths of clinical depression or mental and physical breakdown, to believe that it will produce good seems almost impossible. But it is true, for 'we know that in *all things* God works for *the good* of those who love him, who have been called according to his purpose' (Rom 8:28, italics mine).

Paul was not arguing abstract theology, he was speaking from the depths of experience: the context deals with the problems of suffering and weakness. His words of assurance are echoed down the centuries by countless saints of God from all ages and all conditions and circumstances. God has spoken; many have proved him true in the most dire of situations. *All things* will work together for the *good* of those who are the Lord's people. Once again the exhortation is to tell yourself, out loud if necessary, *that it is true*, despite the way you feel in your depression and despair.

Thus recovery will not be a return to the treadmill unless we make it so – in which case we shall not have learnt our lesson properly. It will be the first rung on a new, specially designed ladder, which will lead us into richer, fuller, more serene service as we climb it rung by rung, in obedience to the Lord who brought us low and has now raised us up. Looking back we shall still shudder at the pain, but we shall not regret the experience, because the Lord will have transformed our lives through it. We shall *know* the difference, even if our work in the church and out of it seems on the surface to be much the same kind of activity as before, for the transformation will be of our inmost self, and our relationship to God. That will make the vital difference, for in a new way our service will spring from:

> 'A heart resigned, submissive, meek,
> My dear Redeemer's throne,
> Where only Christ is heard to speak,
> Where Jesus reigns alone.'

Our only regret will be that we did not learn it before.

14
Helping the broken

Many of us will know individuals who have been broken by the treadmill. Our relationships with them are often bewildering and confusing, for we are not sure what to do and say. Clearly we are not qualified in any way to treat the person concerned. There are, however, a number of things we can do, and a number of others which it is wise to avoid at all costs.

Be encouraging

In the previous chapter we looked at ways in which the broken person can help himself. A principal function of the helper must always be to encourage the positive attitudes outlined there.

Reinforce the certainty of the presence of God, and the assurance that in due time the valley *will* be passed through and left behind. Where possible, actually share in the therapeutic activities which can help so much – the hobbies laid aside long ago, for example. Avoid any reinforcement of negative attitudes or actions. However slight, these must be shunned completely.

Above all be natural, be yourself. Any insincere attempt to be bright and breezy when that is not your natural character will be seen for the hollow sham it is, and will hinder rather than help. The depressive does not need cheering up. He needs practical help. If you yourself are depressed then perhaps you should not consider visiting others in the same condition, for it may be bad for both of you. A genuine, sincere smile and a kind, optimistic demeanour can work wonders. There may be no obvious response, but the impact will be there. The broken one needs to know that you *care*, and that is achieved more by your general natural demeanour than by anything in particular that is consciously *done* or said.

Above all, never give the impression, even by the slightest hint, that having a sick mind is in some way less real than suffering from a sick body. Depression is as real as angina or appendicitis. Similarly, never entertain the thought that depression and stress illnesses are in some way less excusable than so-called physical illness. If you do think this, it will show in your manner and attitude, and be a hindrance to the Lord's using you as a factor in his healing.

We have suggested that in some cases healing may be inhibited by hidden sin or bitterness against others in the depressed and stressed. Discernment of this, I believe, can be achieved only by someone with considerable experience of this kind of counselling, who knows a great deal about the background and history of the person concerned, and then receives the gift of discernment and particular knowledge from the Holy Spirit.

The clear word of God by his Spirit will be necessary before even that person dares take it upon himself to confront the sick one. His knowledge is, anyway, much more likely to drive him to agonized prayer before the Lord, than to immediate and direct confrontation. So never take such a responsibility upon yourself.

If, in your contact, you begin to suspect such a 'root of bitterness', then go to someone of maturity and discernment who knows both you and the sick person well, and reveal it to him in the very strictest confidence. Such a person must be someone whom both you *and* the broken one *trust*. Here again we come back to the need for true spiritual direction – both for you and the broken one.

Don't preach

For a broken Christian the offering of pious advice, however scriptural, will not help at all. He will know it already. And advice like, 'Try to pull yourself together'; or 'What you need is to tell me all about it'; or 'You must just see that things are not really as bad as they seem'; or 'All you need to do is to open yourself to God's Spirit and you will be healed', is not only useless and empty, but likely to be positively harmful.

Just as you have no authority of your own to go to someone with a broken leg and say, 'Get up and walk!' – only the Lord has that right – so you have no authority to say to the depressed and stressed, 'Snap out of it!' That belongs, just as much, to the Lord. The clinically depressed person in himself is just as incapable of snapping out of it as is the man with a broken leg of getting up and walking. For either to take place requires the normal attentions of medical practice, or a miraculous intervention by the Lord.

Sometimes an appropriate course of action is to read to the person short passages of scripture which either emphasize the greatness, faithfulness and love of the Lord, *or* which may awaken a sense of solidarity with a Bible character who expresses the feelings of despair and desparation which the depressed and stressed themselves feel. Do not comment, still less attempt an exposition. The word will speak for itself. The aim is to direct the eye of the mind and heart upwards to God, and to establish empathy between the Bible character and the broken one. God will do this by his Spirit, without our direct intervention. Sometimes there will be an opportunity to comment; but wait until the Lord gives it, and then be brief.

Be prepared to listen

Sometimes the depressed person will want to talk, unprompted. The visitor's job then is simply to listen, and gently to encourage the broken one to pour out the feelings of frustration, anger, despair and bitterness, even to tears. This will provide a deep emotional and psychological release which can only be good, and contribute to healing.

All the negative feelings may be released against *you*; in which case, absorb them and turn the burden over on to the Lord. They may well be feelings against God anyway; if they are overtly so, then so much the better. He understands, he can take it, and to him 'belong mercies and forgivenesses', (Daniel 9:9 AV) – note the plural. Do not try to defend God, he doesn't need our help. In our crucified and risen Lord we have a high priest who not only understands our weaknesses, but also is quite able to absorb our anger and frustration, especially in situations of deep distress. Be prepared to hear the same things often, for one outburst is rarely a sufficient release, and the depressed person will often not remember that he has poured himself out in that way to you before.

The converse of this is being prepared simply to sit in silence for long periods. Almost always you will have to wait for a response to any contribution you make. Even your simple presence means something important – that you care. Don't be discouraged that your being there seems to make no difference to the one who is depressed. Silence is not wasted time.

We also need to be prepared to talk about quite inconsequential and seemingly unimportant things and events. Just the desire to converse can be a sign of progress. We are not there to be sombre and serious and spiritual: we are there to care and share. Much of life consists in apparently inconsequential and unimportant things, and visiting the depressed and stressed is intended to help them return to life in *all* its dimensions – not just to help to right deep psychological wounds. We seek a restoration to wholeness, including the supposedly trivial and insignificant. Attempts to concentrate on the issues we consider important from our perspective, and even on the issues which really are fundamental, can frequently increase the burden, rather than lightening it.

Be constant in prayer

Pray, and keep on praying, before, during and after every visit. Learn to commit every moment silently to the Lord whose representative you are in that situation. Of course, pray for the healing of the one whom you visit, but pray through every act and every sentence and phrase that is spoken; use the silences to turn to the Lord. Not only will such perseverance in prayer serve to prevent mistakes, but it will also ensure that even the mistakes you make will be used for ultimate good. Remember that in *all things* God works for the good for those who love him – and *you* love him, and the *one you are visiting* loves him too, however hidden that love may be at the time of depression.

Pray not only for the one whom you visit, but also for yourself. You need the constant support of the Lord in the taxing, exhausting task he has given you; you need to draw on his love, wisdom, grace and strength to enable you to do his work. Prayer is therefore indispensable. Pray and go on praying.

Work as a member of the local congregation of God's people

You do not exist as a single, isolated, individual Christian; you are a limb of the body of Christ, reaching out to the needy person you are visiting. You are not alone; not only is Christ with you by his Spirit, but the other members of the body are with you also. They have their part to play. The local expression of that body is the church to which you belong. Seek their support, especially in prayer, and pre-eminently at the regular meeting for corporate intercession. There is no need to reveal confidences; a general report on progress and an opening up of your own feelings and problems will result in your being borne up on the wings of the prayers of the saints.

Be prepared to seek and take the advice of other Christians who have greater experience. Do not neglect, either, the expertise of those professionally qualified in psychiatry and counselling. These are dimensions of a true 'whole body' ministry in the local congregation which are perhaps often neglected.

As the visitor to the broken Christian, you are the vital link between that hurt member of the body and your home church. You are therefore essential, however inadequate and unsuccessful you may feel yourself to be. Clearly, one function of such a link will be to encourage the broken saint to come to worship, to hear the word of God and to participate in the Lord's Supper. That may require practical steps to facilitate it, like actually calling for the person to take him to church. Be prepared for him to refuse, even if he has previously agreed. Accept the refusal with a gentle word of encouragement, but do not cajole or try to argue, still less reprimand. Invite the person again; eventually you will receive a promise to come which will actually be kept.

Keep up the link in practical ways too, for many who are depressed and stressed have a mortal fear of being with other people in large numbers, even in church. Provide the church magazine or newsletter regularly, and books and magazines, not necessarily spiritual or improving ones! If your church has a tape ministry then use that too, especially if whole services and not just sermons are recorded. Sermons and convention addresses may well have a place by themselves. But taken out of the context of the complete worship of the whole people of God, they can too easily seem to be lectures pointing the finger at the broken Christian as he listens by himself to a challenge from the word of God. Those who are depressed and stressed take to themselves very easily the condemnatory parts of scripture, without finding comfort and hope in other parts. So a diet of sermons can make them worse rather than better. Set in the context of a full worship service, however, the effect is to draw them subconsciously into the worship of God's people by a process of recall. If the sermons alone are all that is available, choose them wisely. Tapes of singing and praise can also play a part.

It is sometimes a good idea to listen to the tape with the person when you visit; but he may not want that. If so, then simply leave the cassette. Do not leave it too long if it has not been listened to, though. Take it away, and let a few weeks pass before you try another one. The content of the tape itself is not as important as the link it provides with the local company of God's people.

Persevere

It is difficult to exaggerate the discouragements and disappointments that accompany this kind of visiting. Sometimes healing and wholeness return quite quickly, and often suddenly. More often, in my experience, visit follows visit, and there is no perceptible improvement or encouragement. It is easy to give up. Months, even years, may pass without any sign of change. Even if there is change, very often recovery is a matter of peaks and troughs, often high peaks and deep troughs.

Remember what you have taken on. You have chosen to climb off your ladder temporarily (and only rats on ladders have a real ministry in this) in order to get down into the bottom corner of the cage to get alongside a terrified, exhausted and broken rat who has fallen off the treadmill. You have been called to learn to weep with one who is weeping, inwardly if not outwardly. That is a difficult and demanding ministry for anyone. We find it far easier to rejoice with those who rejoice – especially if we have not succumbed to stress and depression ourselves. If we are already subject to depressive tendencies it will still be hard, for we shall have to watch that we don't begin to slide back and change our weeping with someone else into weeping for ourselves.

If things get too much for us then we need to hand over to someone else, preferably someone with more experience and knowledge. To give up in that way is not defeat; it is to admit the magnitude of the problem and to acknowledge that we have done our part. What we have done will not be wasted in the economy of God; and we must be content to be simple links in a chain which is being forged by the Lord himself.

We are always eager to see quick results – in every area of Christian service! But God created time and he uses it. His pace of working is always right, and we must be content to be used by him in simple obedience to the guidance and promptings of his Spirit, through and out of the word of God. Our Lord saved and healed his people by descending to the dirtiest, most depressing, stressful corner of the cage, hanging over the gate of hell itself – which could not stand up against his assault on it. He gives his victory to us, and in this ministry we are permitted in his grace to share in his sufferings to some small degree. Let us never underestimate that privilege. But neither let us make light of the cost to us of such a ministry.

15
Helping non-Christians and lapsed Christians

Many non-Christians break under the strain of the worldly treadmill, and we have a responsibility and ministry to them too. Much of the foregoing practical advice applies to our relationships with them but there are a couple of warnings which need to be added.

First, contact with a broken non-Christian, or even a lapsed one, is not to be seen as a God-given opportunity to preach the 'gospel'. The gospel has to become flesh in us before we can truly communicate it to others. It is communicated by what we are, by what we do and by what we say.

In dealing with the depressed and broken who do not know Christ we have to earn the right to speak, and then only as the Holy Spirit gives us opportunity. We need to allow ourselves to be instruments of *God's* healing. That is achieved only by the love of Christ shining through us, transforming the ordinary acts of kindness in which we engage into the acts of the loving heart and hands of Jesus. We underestimate the power of Christian love in itself. We think that words are always necessary to communicate Christ; they are not. On many occasions they are a hindrance. Let Christ by his love *in* you speak *through* you.

Opportunities to speak will come. They need to be taken, but wisely and with tact and circumspection. Sometimes the experiences of Christians who have been through similar experiences may be used. If discreetly introduced, the broken person may find something there to indentify with, and be gently led on by the Spirit from that point. Even the experiences of biblical characters may find an echo which God can use.

The broken person who makes no Christian profession needs to be loved and wooed into the kingdom. This takes time, and the patience, wisdom and discernment which only Christ can give. It is strange that we take so much care in wooing and courting the one we love in order to eventually be joined in marriage, and how little care we take in allowing Jesus to woo and court someone into a love affair with himself through us. If he has been real during our care of the stressed and depressed non-Christian, then we may well have earned the opportunity for straight speaking when the depression has been cured and the stress problem solved. After all there can be no marriage without a proposal at some time in the relationship! When that proposal is opportune the Lord will, I believe, show us. We are called to follow him, not to walk a step in front. Once again the image of being just one link in a chain being forged by the Lord can be helpful.

It may be that the non-Christian will ask all sorts of questions which provide an opportunity to speak of Jesus and his love. As with Christians, anger and frustration may be directed against God. At least that may be a recognition of God's existence and interest, and that can be pointed out in a kindly way. There is no need to get involved in arguments defending God; he is well able to look after himself. Long intellectual arguments will not necessarily bring the non-Christian any closer to a living relationship with the Lord Jesus. Once again divine discernment is essential.

Above all, the whole must be underpinned by prayer – ours and that of the church. In that situation we are still a limb of the body reaching out to someone in need in the love of Christ. Let us be content to allow him to use us as he wills. It is the simplest and safest way – but probably the most difficult, because it hurts our pride to be so submissive and inconspicuous.

Epilogue

The writing of this book has inevitably involved the reliving of painful experiences and the relearning of hard lessons. It is appropriate, therefore, to conclude by stating some general principles which need to be taken seriously by all Christians, whether susceptible to stress and pressure or not.

I am convinced that our problems with pressure and stress today spring ultimately from four deficiencies in our Christian life, both individual and corporate.

First: our view of God is too small, and we do not *know* what he is really like. Second: the excessive individualism of much Christian thinking and action, and the complementary failure to realize the importance of the Christian community. Third: the fact that we have a false view of the world in which we live, for we don't realize how deeply pagan it is – the former director of Christian Aid, Charles Elliott, calls it 'neo-pagan'. Fourth: we mistake hyperactivity in Christian work for the true life of the Spirit. We rarely experience the richness of the life of God in his people.

Breakdown is not always the result of an unsatisfactory lifestyle, or of attitudes for which the individual is solely responsible. It cannot be completely avoided simply by changing these things. Heredity, personality, earlier history – particularly in childhood and adolescence – illness, bereavement, divorce, pregnancy, the menopause and so on, are all potent factors in the syndrome. We are also caught up in social, work, family and church structures over which we have very little control. So we cannot necessarily avoid reaching breaking-point; but we can begin to examine ourselves and the way we live, to change what we can, and pray that together we may change some of the structures which imprison us.

Our view of God

Our knowledge of what God is like is built over the years
by the traditional disciplines of the Christian life. Too often
those who have proclaimed their evangelicalism most loudly
have emphasized the importance of conversion to the extent
of obscuring the subsequent life of self-discipline which is
part of the proper response to the grace of God in Christ.

The Christian is called to work out in practice the implications of what he already is in Christ (see Romans 6–8).
This involves the systematic study of the scriptures,
working them into the fabric of our personalities, our
thought and life, by prayer and fasting. Thus they become
part of our experience. This discipline is the real 'practice
of the presence of God'.

I discovered the gem of Christian spirituality which has
that title after my own breakdown, when my brothers and
I went through my father's library after his death. It was a
minute pocket edition, only seven by ten cm., and five mm.
thick, but how I regret not having found it years before!
The fact that this slim volume is still in print shows that it
meets a deep need. We all need to put into practice Brother
Lawrence's simple, yet profound, disciplines: 'Our sancti-
fication', he says, 'does not depend upon some alteration in
what we do, but in *doing for God what we commonly do for
ourselves*'; and it is, 'enormous self-deception to believe that
the time of prayer must be different from any other. We
are equally bound to be one with God by what we do in
times of action as by the time of prayer at its special hour.'
(Brother Lawrence, *The Practice of the Presence of God*
trans. E. M. Blaiklock; London: Hodder and Stoughton,
1981, p.29. Italics mine.)

The presence of God must pervade every part of our
lives; that can be achieved only by self-discipline inspired,
sustained and used by the grace of God, by his Spirit.

Recognition of the Christian community

The real, intelligent and prayerful support of the Christian community of which we are a part can only be realized by practice and discipline. 'Community' does not just materialize when we need it most; it has to be developed as a normal part of Christian growth. This means the costly building of deep relationships *now*. Certainly in far too many local churches the structures militate against and inhibit, rather than further, the growth of such essential links. They need to change. However, there is still much that we can do without drastic change, but only at the cost of sacrificing a substantial part of the hyperactivity which often passes for the service of God.

The community itself also needs to learn – and *we* are that community – not to treat mental breakdown and succumbing to stress as spiritual defeats. As I said in the last chapter, even if we do not say so, the fact that we *think* so will be apparent in our behaviour, and will be sensed by anyone to whom we try to minister. Even if it were true that breakdown was such a defeat, and it is not necessarily so, then let us remind ourselves that we, too, have areas of spiritual defeat in our lives – the only difference is that ours are not so unavoidably public.

We tend to *assume* that repentance is needed – even if it is we do not *know* so – and our support may thus be qualified or tinged with condemnation. But the only attitude of mind and heart which is of any value in such situations is sheer persevering, unqualified, active love. That is an attitude we need to cultivate generally in the body of Christ (1 Cor 13:4–8a); it cannot be put on when the special need arises. Such love comes only because the Lord first loved us, and only as we let his love flow into our personalities by practising his presence both individually and corporately.

A realistic perception of our society

The third dimension of realism that needs to come into our thinking relates to the society in which we live. Our society is utterly man-centred. Our modern knowledge of the vastness and complexity of the universe has, supposedly, removed the earth from the centre of things. It is reputed to have demonstrated the utter insignificance of man. In practice, however, man is more at the centre of his intellectual universe than he ever was when he believed that this small planet was the centre of the universe. We Christians need to remember that, for we live in an intellectual, psychological and spiritual world which is totally dependent upon God. The only basis for *real* manward relations is found in a God-centred orientation of our whole being.

If we are oriented towards God at the deepest levels of our being, then it must show in our Christian community and its relationships and actions. Conformity to and compromise with the world outside is all too easy; the devil sees to that. Society will be transformed only as the leaven of holy love, present in power in the Christian community, permeates outwards through its members in the places, geographical and vocational, in which God has set them. It is his plan and strategy, not ours, that matters. All truly Christian social and political action will spring from the worship and prayer of the local Christian community, as part of the wider church of Christ.

Perhaps one of the areas of witness in the world today is in this area of pressure and stress. As Christians we should be able to turn the treadmill into the ladder, and cope with the rat race and its associated evils by putting it into its proper perspective. Our frame of reference is different; we know the One who is in full control of the cage and all its inhabitants; he sees every treadmill, and provides every ladder. He knows the true position of every rat, both Christian and non-Christian. Brother Lawrence again hits the nail on the head:

'Think often of God, day and night, in all your tasks, in all your religious duties, even in all your amusements. He is always at your side. Do not fail in fellowship with him. You would consider it discourteous to neglect a friend who visited you. Why abandon God and leave him alone? Do not then forget him. Think of him often. Worship him all the time. Live and die with him. That is the Christian's lovely task, in a word, our calling. If we do not know it we must learn it.'   (p.53)

The pressures of contemporary life are such that some will break, however well prepared they are. Our faithfulness to God will then be seen in the way we cope with breakdown – in ourselves, should it come to us, and in others to whom we are bound in the fellowship of Christ's church. God may choose to test our faith in this particular way. Not, as we have seen, to prove to *him* how strong it is, but to show us, and thereby to increase our faith and fit us for greater and more responsible tasks in the service of his kingdom.

Those who have been brought low in mental and physical breakdown can rise to new heights of service and reach deeper levels of trust through their affliction. This can still be so, even though they may have brought it on themselves. No one is so low that he cannot be raised again to fresh and unimagined levels of active service for the Lord. No one is so broken that he cannot experience and exercise a more profound faith and knowledge of the Lord as a result.

Hyperactivity or the work of the Spirit?

Restoration and rehabilitation depend not only upon the individual, but upon the local Christian community who help him. Too often such communities are hampered in this ministry by the hyperactivity they have confused with true church life. As we have seen, such activity is often the *cause* of the breakdown in the first place! We need to recover a vision in the church of what real spiritual life means: worship in word and sacrament, and in prayer, both individual and corporate. Everything which comes from that will be effective because it will spring from the promptings of the Holy Spirit, not from a carnal desire to do something for God, which can so easily turn into something I do for myself. How I long for the church of the living God to get her priorities right, and to have the courage to *set* them right when the real issues are grasped and faced. We shall then have fewer sick and weak rats, and our efforts will be devoted to climbing the ladder of glory rather than in keeping the ecclesiastical treadmill turning.

Those who do not know the Lord see the cage only from the inside; for them the treadmill can never become a ladder. Even if they reach the very top of the worldly treadmill their fall in the end is quite inevitable, so that ultimately all end up at the bottom of the cage. They have no resources from outside. Some come to terms with the mill, particularly those who either get higher than most, or who succeed in finding a not too strenuous part of the mill. Others settle for the bottom of the cage anyway, and reflect on the cage and the mill without too much pressure. But they have no hope of getting out. Their whole world is still the cage.

What a tragedy it is that so many Christians turn God's ladder into a treadmill in their own individual lives! How sad that so many churches turn what should be the joyful, fulfilling service of the Lord into another treadmill which must be kept going at all costs! The Lord forgive and save us from ourselves – and from our churches. May he teach us the way of true piety and real service that brings glory to the name of the Lord and *thus* blessing to those who engage in it.

Let Brother Lawrence have the last word:

'Let us give our thoughts completely to knowing God. The more one knows him, the more one wants to know him, and since love is measured commonly by knowledge, then, the deeper and more extensive knowledge shall be, so love will be the greater, and, if love is great, we shall love him equally in suffering and consolation.

Let us not hold ourselves back by seeking or loving God for the favours he bestows upon us, lofty though they can be, or for those he can do for us. These favours, great though they are, will never bring us as near to him as faith does by one simple act. Let us seek him often through this virtue. He is in our midst. Let us seek him nowhere else. Are we not discourteous and guilty of ignoring him, busying ourselves with a thousand trifles which displease, and perhaps which offend him? He endures them all the same, but it is much to be feared that one day they may cost us dearly.

Let us begin by being his without reservation. Let us banish from heart and mind all that which is not himself. He wants to be the only one. Ask of him this grace. If we do, on our part, what we can, we shall soon see the change for which we hope.'   (pp.62 – 63)

Further Reading

I am diffident about recommending books to those who have already reached breaking-point, for two reasons.

First, each breakdown is that of an individual, and though there are general principles which underlie much depression and stress, in my experience each individual needs personal attention tailored to his or her quite personal, even unique, needs.

Second, if a broken Christian reads a book which promises to enable him to overcome the stress and depression provided he takes certain steps, and having read it, the promise is not fulfilled, then his latter situation is far worse than the first. In my experience, the promise of cure is often *not* fulfilled, and the depressed person feels an even greater sense of failure and guilt.

Furthermore, both my wife and myself, who have passed through the valley of the shadow which can be touched, have found that the only real help comes from scripture, particularly the psalms. This is perhaps not surprising if the scriptures are indeed the word of God to man. So my advice to those who have been broken is to concentrate on scripture. This, with a good, amusing novel as light reading, will probably be as much help as a dozen books which promise a cure. So the list of books which follows is really intended for those who have not yet been brought low, or who want to help those who have been broken by the mill.

The list is by no means exhaustive. I am not prepared to recommend books which I have not read, and I have read only a small fraction of those available. Some of those I have read I would not recommend on any account – but it would be churlish to produce a list of books to avoid at all costs! Inevitably, the list is highly personal since it is the product of reactions and judgments which stem from individual experience. Nevertheless, it may be of some help. The books are listed alphabetically by author, with occasional comments. Those which are now out of print are well worth looking out for in the 'second-hand' departments of book shops.

Sir Norman Anderson, An Adopted Son: the Story of my Life.
(Leicester, IVP, 1985.) This moving autobiography faithfully records the reactions of an eminent Christian and his wife to the traumas encountered in the course of an exciting and

eventful life. It includes their reactions to the loss of their three children as young adults, in the space of five years. All three were committed Christians, and showed extreme promise in their separate careers.

Michael Baughen, The Prayer Principle. (London, Mowbray, 1983.) An eminently readable, practical and challenging consideration of all the dimensions of prayer in both personal and corporate Christian living. Since prayer is the core of worship, serious study of the issues raised in the book is of basic importance in the examination of our personal lives and the corporate life of the church to which we belong.

E M Blaiklock, Between the Sunset and the Stars: coming to terms with old age. (London, Hodder and Stoughton, 1982.) Towards the end of a long life, an eminent servant of the Lord reflects on the problems, possibilities and hopes of old age. Invaluable as an insight into the thoughts and reactions of the old, reflected on from the perspective of a Christian and the unique hope which is his.

L J Crabbe, Basic Principles of Biblical Counselling: showing care in the local church. (Basingstoke, Marshalls, 1985.) The paperback version of an earlier edition published in 1975. I have found it helpful in defining aims and analysing individual problems from a biblical perspective. It is designed for the Christian layman, not the professional. Its aim is not to provide a 'method' or technique, but to help the reader to think through the counselling framework in the local church. It takes both clergy and lay involvement into account.

L J Crabbe, Effective Biblical Counselling: how to become a capable counsellor. (Basingstoke, Marshalls, 1985.) The paperback version of the 1977 edition. This is a follow-up to the previous volume, expanding and developing some of the ideas set out there. Despite its title and, to a degree, its approach, it should *not* be used as a textbook to solve all the stress and depression problems in the congregation.

Selwyn Hughes, Seven Steps to Overcoming Depression. (Basingstoke, Marshalls, 1982.) This is a short and clear examination of the problems of depression in Christians. It might work for some suffering from depression, and indeed in Mr Hughes' experience it clearly has worked for a large number. In my experience some depressions are much too complicated to yield to this rather simplistic approach. It is more a book to enable the ordinary Christian to gain some understanding of depression.

Frank Lake, Tight Corners in Pastoral Counselling. (London, Darton Longman and Todd, 1981). This is a book for the pastor and specialist counsellor. It is written by the founder of the Clinical Theology movement, and from that perspective. Wider in scope than the area of stress and depression, it is useful, if somewhat technical.

Brother Lawrence, The Practice of the Presence of God. (Trans and introduced by E M Blaiklock; London, Hodder and Stoughton, 1981.) The one book on the list which should be read by everyone, whether or not they are, or have been, broken. It cannot be recommended too highly, for it gets to the root of the problem.

C S Lewis, A Grief Observed. (London, Faber and Faber, 1960.) The poignant and brutally honest record of the author's reactions to the terminal illness and death of his wife. He articulates the deepest feelings not only of many bereaved people, but also of many in deep depression; they, too, are suffering a form of self-bereavement. The BBC film, *Shadowlands*, produced by Norman Stone, himself a committed Christian, brilliantly re-creates the situation and the reactions. Neither, I think, should be used for those in a state of depression, because the result might be even deeper depression. But Lewis' book is compulsory reading for all who would seek to understand how depressed people feel, as a preparation for helping and counselling.

D M Lloyd-Jones, Spiritual Depression: its causes and cure. (London, Pickering and Inglis, 1965.) This exhaustive biblical study is very much for the theologically minded. I think that few individuals actually in the depths of depression would be able to tackle it. For the theologically minded it must be essential reading.

Edith Schaeffer, Affliction. (London, Hodder and Stoughton, 1973.) A helpful and compassionate study of suffering in the Christian's life, including stress-related illnesses and depression. It might be especially helpful to those who, having been broken, ask, 'Why should it happen to me?'

William Still, Rhythms of Rest and Work. (Aberdeen, Didasko Press, no date. Obtainable from 18 Morningside Gardens, Aberdeen, AB1 7NS: price 65p + postage.) This booklet is an examination of the peace which Christ brings, in its spiritual, psychological and physical outworking in the Christian life. It is both profound in its understanding of scripture and highly practical in its application of it. The value of this little-known booklet can hardly be overestimated. The proof of its worth might be the fact that its author is still actively ministering at the age of seventy-five in his own congregation, fulfilling the commitments of a diary which would cause many men half his age to blanch!

Anne J Townsend, Suffering without Pretending. (London, Scripture Union, 1980.) Now out of print, this is a valuable book which treats the problem of suffering realistically at a number of levels. It contains much practical wisdom purged in the furnace of personal experience.

Paul Tournier, A Place for You. (Trans E Hudson, 1968; Crowborough, Highland Books.) The mature reflection of a Christian doctor who has extensive and profound experience of personal counselling, both inside and outside the church. It is very relevant to the problems which are our main concern.

Paul Tournier, Escape from Loneliness. (Trans W L Jenkins, 1962; Crowborough, Highland Books.) A masterly and practical analysis of the reasons why, even in the whirl of contemporary social and church activity, there is a fundamental loneliness in the hearts of so many. The analysis concludes that there is a necessity for real, practical commitment to Jesus Christ.

Evelyn Underhill, The Spiritual Life. (Oxford, Mowbury, 1984.) This book of practical devotion was written from a Catholic perspective in 1937. It contains much to help the ordinary

Christian along the road to balance and equanimity through his relationship to his Lord, which is given as the best antidote to stress and pressure. Its advice can be a great help in keeping rats on the ladder.

David Watson, Discipleship. (London, Hodder and Stoughton, 1981.) A standard manual for Christian disciples. It asks many hard and pertinent questions about what it means to be on the ladder of discipleship in our western world today.

John White, The Masks of Melancholy: a Christian psychiatrist looks at depression and suicide. (Leicester, IVP, 1982.) Probably the best study of depression written from the perspective of the evangelical Christian. It is essential reading for all who aspire to help and counsel depressives in any profound way, but probably not a book to give to someone who is in a state of depression.

R E O White, A Guide to Pastoral Care. (London, Pickering and Inglis, 1976.) A general manual of pastoral care which deals with a wide range of personal problems, including depression and stress. It is very valuable for its extensive bibliographies, which should provide an excellent starting point for anyone who wishes to pursue the various topics to a more profound level. Probably not for the general helper, but rather more use to the person who has a real gift for counselling at the personal level, and wishes to develop it for the Lord's use.

Olive Wyon, The School of Prayer. (London, SCM, 1950.) This book which is unfortunately now out of print, has proved a great help to me in my climb up the ladder of discipleship. It deserves to stand alongside the great classics of Christian spirituality. It is the most helpful book on prayer that I know, for it is intensely practical as well as intensely spiritual. If you can lay your hands on a copy, then read it, learn it, and inwardly digest it so as to make it part of your practical, mental and spiritual apparatus.

APPENDIX A: Sunday worship

In my original draft, discussing the priority of worship I wrote that I believed Christians on the ladder should be twice at worship on a Sunday, if at all possible. I said that only reasons which would stand up to the scrutiny of a holy God who knows all the secrets of our hearts were sufficient to excuse our absence. It was thought that I was really being too hard and inflexible in putting things so strongly. On reflection I agreed and the draft was changed for the better, for I have no desire to induce unwarranted guilt feelings in any of my readers. My original statements, however, had two deep convictions behind them.

The first is that far too many apparently keen Christians sit too easily on their attendance at the central acts of the body of Christ. Their reasons are often quite insubstantial. Excuses which they wouldn't dare make to their parents to avoid visiting them seem to be considered quite adequate to offer to God as reasons for not attending his house to worship with his people. Truancy from the house of God is considered more excusable than truancy from school! Yet which ultimately is more important? It is our *actions* that reveal where our real priorities lie.

The second conviction is that the Christian community has become deeply infected by a false emphasis on the individual which derives more from the specious philosophies rooted in the Enlightenment than in the revealed truth given in scripture. Evangelicals have been particularly prone to the infection, and are now reaping the consequences in many areas of church life – including a disturbingly high incidence of stress, breakdown and depression. We need to recover the vision of the family of God, the pilgrim people of God, and the body of Christ as a visible entity in this world. That family, people and body is created by God with a view to its being, *corporately*, the bride of Christ, offering itself in perfect worship to him eternally. The community is primarily a *worshipping* community, and from that worship flows all else that is of God. This surely can be traced through the New Testament, both in its own distinctiveness, and in its reference to and dependence upon the Old. Ephesians and Colossians especially have such an emphasis, as does Revelation, but the idea is present almost everywhere in scripture. This is not to deny the importance of the individual, but rather to put the individual and his role in a fully biblical context. Corporate worship must be the central activity of the people of God here on earth. And *corporate* includes everyone who is in any way committed, together with their families.

To insist on this is not to imply that our present ways of organizing the times and content of our acts of worship are satisfactory, still less ideal and unalterable. Serious thought needs to be given to our traditional patterns of twice on Sunday and once or twice midweek, and whether they any longer meet the requirement for the primacy of worship in the most effective way. But we shall only think these issues through when we begin to recognize our *true* priorities, and work outwards in our thinking from the centrality of corporate worship in the life of the people of God.

APPENDIX B:
Towards a personal check-up

The following suggestions are intended to help anyone who wishes to attempt an appraisal of their personal balance of life. Such an exercise can be very revealing. To be of any real help, of course, it is necessary to try to be totally honest, and not fudge answers to suit what we would like to come out! If at all possible, the appraisal should be done with the help of a close friend.

STEP ONE
During a normal fortnight of your ordinary life, keep a diary of what you do in every half-hour of every day.

If you can, continue it for a month. This can best be done by making out a chart which is divided into forty-eight separate sections for each day (ie forty-eight half-hour slots). An ordinary, ruled A4 sheet usually contains thirty-two spaces between the ruled lines; if the top twenty-four spaces are used, and a dividing line is ruled down the centre of the page, the necessary forty-eight spaces are created, and there is room at the bottom for a subsequent review of the information recorded. The two columns are each then subdivided into two, providing a left column in which to write the starting time of each half-hour, and a right one in which the activity for that half-hour can be recorded. In recording the time it is best to use the 24–hour clock (ie midnight is 0000 hours, 6 am is 0600, 10 am is 1000, noon is 1200, 5 pm is 1700, 10 pm is 2200, and so on); this saves possible confusion. One sheet then serves for one day. The day and date should be written at the top of the sheet as the diary is kept. If you have access to a photocopier the task of making the required number of sheets is made much easier.

In keeping the diary be as precise as possible in your recording. It is not, of course, necessary to record activities as they are undertaken, which is often very inconvenient; but they should be recorded as soon as possible after they occur. Leaving too much for later on will inevitably lead to an incomplete or, worse still, an invented diary, which will destroy the purpose of the exercise.

Keeping the diary is a discipline which is valuable in itself, but its purpose is to aid self-analysis. That is why night-time is not excluded. It is necessary to record not only the time you go to bed, but also the time you go to sleep, and any periods of wakefulness during the night. Clearly, the time you go to sleep will be recorded the next morning, and will probably be somewhat approximate too! The real concern is to find out whether you consistently take a long time to go to sleep. Wakeful periods need not be measured unless they are long, in which case you will usually be *very* conscious of the time period. But even a note to indicate that your sleep was broken two or three times during the night will help the examination of the record. The time you wake is also important, particularly if it is followed by a period of restlessness, or even turmoil, before you actually rise.

While the diary will be mainly concerned with your activities, it can also be helpful to record how you actually feel at particular times – pressured by the activity, or relaxed; whether it is a burden and effort, or easily performed; enjoyable or distasteful, and so on. There are other details which may have significance, and which may be recorded if the diary can be kept private and personal. For example, if you are married, you may wish to note when you actually express affection to your wife or husband by an embrace or a more than formal kiss, and in more intimate ways. Indeed, should you run the diary for a second period, it is possible on the basis of the experience of the first period to work out a symbolic code to indicate feelings and reactions, and intimacies of various kinds. For those not married, it is useful to record the degree of friendship expressed in various contacts and social occasions. In all relatively close relationships it can be useful to record those occasions when there are differences of opinion, even rows.

The whole point of the diary is to enable you to look at yourself and your lifestyle as objectively as possible, not with morbid, self-condemnatory introspection, but with a view to working towards the changes which will almost certainly be indicated by the appraisal. Nor is the diary intended to stimulate guilt feelings. Its purpose is solely factual and analytical, which is why complete honesty in its recording is an absolute necessity.

STEP TWO

Calculate the time spent each week on the various activities noted down.

This has two parts:

1. Divide the activities into categories.

The basic categories might be:

Work

This would include our paid employment, or the work we do as our normal routine. For example a wife and mother would include the time spent in domestic work and caring for the children. Or in a home where both parents work either full-time or part-time, the periods spent sharing domestic chores might be included, though distinguished from the paid employment. All sorts of sub-divisions of the category are possible and perhaps necessary, in accordance with the kind of work we do.

Worship

This category needs sub-division:
- full corporate worship with the whole church;
- family worship, shared with one or more members of the household;
- private worship.

Worship includes prayer and devotional study and reading of the scriptures. Worship and sharing in house-groups forms another sub-category.

Bible study

This cannot always be separated from worship, but I believe that most Christians ought to find some time for study of the scriptures in some depth, apart from their devotional use of the word of God.

Church activities

In this I would include all activities associated with the church which are not included in 'worship' above. Thus Sunday school and Bible class teaching would be put in this group, but family services or family communion would not. Nor would we include here the time spent with the main congregation in churches where the younger members take part in a portion of the services. The time spent out of the main congregation would be included, however. Youth clubs, and other organizations, church committees and the like, all fall under this heading.

Relaxation

This also needs sub-division according to the particular life and calling in which the Lord has led you. It includes time spent with the family and friends in a social way, and corporate social activities in the church or outside it. Sport, watching television, gardening (if it's not simply a chore), DIY (if it's a hobby rather than a necessity which doesn't relax you) may be included here.

Eating

Don't include social meals which are an enjoyment rather than a necessity. Preparation, however, if it is not in itself a relaxing enjoyment, should be included under 'work' as should clearing away and washing up. The point of this is to find out if you are rushing meals in order to do other things considered to be more important.

Travelling

Many of us spend a lot of time travelling, especially to and from work. We can discipline ourselves to use this time profitably, perhaps in reading or prayer, perhaps in other ways. Most of us will be surprised at the amount of time we spend on this activity.

Sleeping

We need to know the amount of time involved here, but more particularly the relation between the time we spend in bed trying to sleep, and the time we actually spend sleeping.

Our lives are individual, and so we can set out only the most basic grouping here. Each of us needs to work out the most useful and effective grouping for our own situation. Once we have developed this we need to stick to it as closely as possible in order to be able to compare later appraisals.

2. Using the diary entries, calculate the time spent in each category.

The result will appear as a number of half-hours. If the exercise has been over two weeks divide these totals by two; if over four weeks, divide by four. This produces a weekly average for each activity.

STEP THREE

Evaluate the proportions of time spent on the various activities in terms of the principles and priorities set out in this book.

In particular, if *Worship* is not significantly larger than *Church activities*, then begin to ask questions about the possible effectiveness of those activities.

If you are engaged in certain *Church activities* that involve teaching, then examine *Bible study* very carefully; they should, perhaps, at least be equal.

If *Work* is very large in proportion to the rest, then perhaps attention needs to be given to that area of your life.

If *Relaxation* is small, or even absent, start asking questions about how it might be increased; but if it is large, especially compared with *Worship* and *Bible study*, then begin to ask whether relaxation has become self-indulgence.

If *Eating* reveals a significant number of rushed meals, ask why, and seek to change.

If, under *Sleeping*, we spend significantly more time in bed trying to sleep than we do actually sleeping, then we need to ask some serious questions. If this is a regular pattern over a period, we need to ask some very serious questions about our lifestyle, and perhaps seek professional advice. If this is coupled with a poor record under *Eating*, then radical reappraisal of our way of life is essential, perhaps with professional help.

If *Travelling* shows up a large amount of time, then we need to ask how we use it.

STEP FOUR
If Step Three reveals a need for change – small, large or drastic – then DO SOMETHING ABOUT IT!

This is not intended to be an exercise in collecting information. It is meant to provide a basis for planned and deliberate change, in order to get more firmly on the ladder at the very least, and to get off the treadmill on to the ladder if a need for really drastic change is indicated. This requires as much determination as weight-watching or keeping fit, and might indeed include both.

STEP FIVE
Repeat Step One after an appropriate interval, and Steps Two to Four if they still prove to be necessary.

Those who have had to undertake a radical reappraisal should assess their changes by means of Step One after three or four months. For those whose changes have been less drastic, six to eight months might be adequate. For those with favourable results, sixteen to eighteen months can elapse before trying Step One again. And for everyone, a check-up after two years might be useful.

Any radical change to one's life pattern, like changing a job, moving house, additions to the family, increased responsibilities at work or in the church, should always be followed by a check-up once the new pattern has become established.

STEP SIX
Repeat the process at regular intervals!